PROMOTING TEAMWORK
IN PRIMARY CARE

PROMOTING TEAMWORK

IN

PRIMARY CARE

A Research-based

Appro

Edited by

Pauline Pea...

Senior Lecturer in Primary Care Nursing,
University of Newcastle upon Tyne,
Newcastle upon Tyne, UK

and

John Spencer

Senior Lecturer in Primary Health Care,
University of Newcastle upon Tyne,
Newcastle upon Tyne, UK

ARNOLD

A member of the Hodder Headline Group
LONDON • SYDNEY • AUCKLAND

First published in Great Britain in 1997 by
Arnold, a member of the Hodder Headline Group,
338 Euston Road, London NW1 3BH

Whilst the advice and information in this book is believed to be true and
accurate at the time of going to press, neither the authors nor the publisher
can accept any legal responsibility or liability for any errors or omissions
that may be made.

British Library Cataloguing in Publication Data
A catalogue record for this book is available from the British Library

Library of Congress Cataloging-in-Publication Data
A catalog record for this book is available from the Library of Congress

ISBN 0 340 65244 6

Composition in 10/12pt Palatino by Phoenix Photosetting, Chatham, Kent
Printed and bound in Great Britain by J W Arrowsmith Ltd, Bristol

Contents

List of contributors

Richard Baker
Richard Baker is Director of the Eli Lilly National Clinical Audit Centre, Department of General Practice and Primary Health Care, University of Leicester. The Centre was set up as a resource for health professionals, health authorities and others in the field of clinical audit or quality assurance. Its principal remit is research into effective methods of audit in primary health care and at the interface between primary and secondary care. Dr Baker also practises as a GP. His research interests include measuring patient satisfaction, developing evidence-based audit protocols for primary care, and the evaluation of methods for implementing change.

Gaynor Bennett
Gaynor Bennett has degrees in psychology and research methods and over 10 years of research experience in university departments and as a freelance. Her principal specialism is in issues of multidisciplinary collaboration in primary care, a subject on which she is finalising a PhD. Her current freelance work includes evaluations of a counselling service and of a clinical psychology service in primary care, as well as a multicultural health project.

Ros Bryar
Since September 1995, Ros Bryar has held a joint post as Professor of Community Healthcare Nursing Practice at the University of Hull and Head of Profession for Health Visiting at Hull and Holderness Community Health NHS Trust. She spends 60 per cent of her time with the Trust, where she has responsibility for the professional development of Health Visiting, and has a small caseload. In the University, she is involved in research supervision and in the work of the Research and Development Division in the School of Health. She spent 10 years in South Wales as a Health Visitor and lecturer, working in Teamcare Valleys and latterly as Co-ordinator of the Diploma in Community Health Studies, Swansea. She qualified as a Health Visitor in 1975 when she completed her nursing degree at Manchester. Her research interests include the transition of practitioner to

researcher, the research base of Health Visiting, and the application of theory to midwifery practice.

Sheila Edward
Sheila Edward is currently working as a Research Associate in the Faculty of Health, Social Work and Education at the University of Northumbria at Newcastle. After a long first career in the National Library of Scotland and the Bodleian Library, she retrained in human resource management and has since worked in a variety of staff development, teaching and research roles, most recently at the Scottish Council for Research in Education. She is currently completing a doctoral thesis on concepts of staff membership, development and practice in multiprofessional settings and is also working on two national projects, on career entry profiling for newly qualified teachers and on preparation for the developing role of the community children's nurse, commissioned by the English Nursing Board.

Debbie Freake
Debbie Freake qualified from Newcastle Medical School in 1987 and trained on the Northumbria Vocational Training Scheme. She is employed by the University of Newcastle upon Tyne as a Lecturer in Primary Health Care, and works as a GP within the Department of Primary Health Care's University Teaching Practice. She takes part in undergraduate and post-graduate teaching and is involved with local service development and locality commissioning.

Susan Gooding
Susan Gooding, health educator, teacher and nurse, was until recently Director of the Health Education Authority (HEA) National Unit for Health Promotion in Primary Care, Oxford. Previously, she was Manager, Trainer and Facilitator of the HEA's Multidisciplinary Team Workshop Programme. She is now Research and Development Nurse for the Wessex Primary Care Research Network, University of Southampton.

Lynne Graver
Lynne Graver is now a lecturer and researcher, having formerly been a nurse, midwife and nurse teacher. She is currently undertaking doctoral research in the development of primary health care at Liverpool John Moores University.

Hilary Hearnshaw
Hilary Hearnshaw was appointed as Lecturer in Clinical Audit at the Eli Lilly National Clinical Audit Centre, Department of General Practice and Primary Health Care, University of Leicester, in 1992. Her previous academic research career had been in psychology ergonomics and

Geographical Information Systems. Her research interests include the fields of behaviour change of clinicians, evaluation of the effectiveness of clinical audit and development of patient evaluation instruments for primary care and interface experiences. She has also been involved in the development and running of software training courses, courses for Primary Care Audit Group chairs, and a university certificate course for clinical audit support staff.

Harriet Hudson

Harriet Hudson is employed by the University of Dundee at the Tayside Centre for General Practice. Her main roles are development of the under-graduate medical curriculum, research into the care of frail elderly people, and general practice development and support using qualitative research methodologies for the basis of change. Her background is in sociology and social administration.

Helen Joesbury

Helen Joesbury is a general practitioner at Woodseats Medical Centre in Sheffield, and a part-time lecturer in the Department of General Practice, University of Sheffield. Her research interests include undergraduate education and curriculum development, and competencies in primary care.

Sarah Long

Sarah Long is a Research Fellow currently working on the Primary Health Care Team Competencies Project in the Department of General Practice, University of Sheffield. Her background is in health visiting. She has completed a Master of Medical Sciences in Primary and Community Care, with a dissertation on teamwork in general practice.

Pauline Pearson

Pauline Pearson is a health visitor and Senior Lecturer in Primary Care Nursing in the Department of Primary Health Care at the University of Newcastle upon Tyne. She previously worked as a researcher, as a community development worker and as a health visitor with four practices. She has had a longstanding interest in interdisciplinary working in primary and community care.

Brenda Poulton

Brenda Poulton is a Research Officer at the Daphne Heald Research Unit, Royal College of Nursing. She undertook doctoral research on effective multidisciplinary teamwork in primary health care at the Institute of Work Psychology, University of Sheffield. Her more recent work has involved a multidisciplinary audit in primary health care project (funded by the NHS Executive), producing a resource on contracting for multidisciplinary team workshop programmes (funded by the Health Education Authority) and an evaluation of practice-based teams for Cardiff Community Trust and Hillingdon Health Authority.

Alice Southern
Alice Southern is a graduate in Information Science who has moved into the field of audit and quality improvement. She has been Audit Facilitator for the North Tyneside Medical Audit Advisory Group for several years, and is now one of two Audit Facilitators for Newcastle and North Tyne Health Authority.

John Spencer
John Spencer is a general practitioner and Senior Lecturer in Primary Health Care in the Department of Primary Health Care at the University of Newcastle. He was very involved in establishing medical audit advisory groups in the North East, was Royal College of General Practitioners Audit Fellow between 1990 and 1993, and a member of Newcastle's Local Organising Team. Much of his research to date has been focused on audit in primary health care.

Paul Thomas
Paul Thomas is a general practitioner and Senior Lecturer in the Department of Primary Health Care and General Practice at Imperial College School of Medicine at St Mary's Hospital Medical School, London. He was formerly Primary Health Care facilitator and Continuing Medical Education tutor in Liverpool where he developed an interest in the use of interdisciplinary learning methods.

Michael West
Michael West is Professor of Work and Organisational Psychology at the Institute of Work Psychology, University of Sheffield, and Co-Director of the Corporate Performance Programme of the Centre for Economic Performance at the London School of Economics. He has authored, edited or co-edited eight books, and written more than 100 articles for scientific and practitioner publications, as well as chapters in scholarly books. His research interests include innovation and creativity at work, team and organisational effectiveness, and mental health at work, with particular reference to NHS organisations.

Tim Usherwood
Tim Usherwood is Professor of General Practice at the University of Sydney. Before moving to Australia he worked in Sheffield, Glasgow and Greenock. His research interests include organisational studies in primary health care, management of depressive illness in the community, and studies in medical education.

Tim van Zwanenberg

Tim van Zwanenberg has wide-ranging experience as a general practitioner in inner-city Newcastle, and as an academic and health services manager. After 6 years as a GP in Newcastle in the 1970s, he worked for nearly 5 years in Papua New Guinea. Back in the UK, he spent another 6 years as a GP and senior lecturer in primary health care in Newcastle before working for a year with the NHS Management Executive in London. In 1992 he became Director of Primary Care for the old Northern Region, taking up post as Director of Health Commissioning and Primary Care Development with Newcastle and North Tyneside Health Authority in 1994. In 1996 he moved to become the first Chair of Postgraduate General Practice at Newcastle University. He has written widely on prescribing, audit and primary care development.

Foreword

It has become a truism to say that health care assumes progressively more complexity. There are two major factors contributing to this. First, the expanded range of skills needed to meet the varied requirements of patients with long-term illness, who are now increasingly drawn from the ageing section of the population, means that more professionals are involved in every case. Secondly, the imperative of seeking cost-effectiveness requires decisions to be built upon a sound scientific base. This book addresses both issues, and thus makes a very important contribution to the literature.

Even if one were to rely upon purely anecdotal evidence, few observers of the health and social services could fail to recognise that most of the unnecessary problems besetting patients occur because of poor communication between the multiplicity of people and disciplines involved. Good teamwork has long been recognised as the solution, but for far too many people it is still honoured more in the breach than in practice.

The troubles start early. Students learn from disciplines separated by departmental boundaries, and observe practitioners who maintain their separate intellectual authoritarianism. As they progress, they will often understand little about the skills and aspirations of other health care workers, and medical students, in particular, are often given to understand that health care is based upon the doctor. Likewise, continuing education and professional development are largely unidisciplinary. Small wonder that attitudes develop which contribute to a fragmentation of care.

Primary care has a better record than most areas for promoting teamwork and seeking to generate more effective practice, but even here the report has to be 'could do better'. There are shining examples of educational initiatives in interprofessional education, examples of imaginative work being done and of studies showing the beneficial effects of teamworking, but these are scattered throughout the literature and not easily accessed. Dr Pearson and Dr Spencer have addressed this difficulty and have gathered a range of contributors with really practical experience of the problems, and the means of overcoming them, drawn from all over the UK.

This brief note does not do justice to the many wise things said in this book, which deserves to be studied by doctors, nurses, social workers and managers. It should be read by students of all of these disciplines, and it should not be confined to those working in primary care, for much that is said is equally pertinent to the secondary care field. The authors have made a real contribution to continuity of care, and thus to improving the service that patients can expect.

Sir Michael Drury
Bromsgrove, 1996

Acknowledgements

We are grateful for the help and support of a wide variety of people in bringing this book to fruition. In particular, we would like to thank the contributors for their enthusiasm and persistence, Margaret Levy, Mary Scott and Anne Corradine for their hard work and good humour through several drafts, and our families and friends for their forbearance over many months.

Pauline Pearson
John Spencer
Newcastle upon Tyne, 1996

1

The primary health care team: an overview

John Spencer

Introduction

The primary health care team has become one of the prevailing concepts of the last decade in the UK health care system. It is part of the rhetoric of the new NHS and, indeed, it is hard to imagine how we shall rise to the challenge of the 'primary care-led NHS' and the new styles of working that are envisaged, without developing multidisciplinary teams that function effectively and efficiently.

Government white papers over the past decade have repeatedly emphasised that primary health care is best delivered by a team of professionals working in a community. Furthermore, this is usually seen as being based around general practice (Jarman and Cumberlege, 1987; Waine, 1992). For instance, in *Choice and Opportunity. Primary Care: The Future* (Secretary of State for Health, 1996) all three of the main objectives of the 'emerging agenda' have major implications for the primary health care team (PHCT). In many respects our ability to 'deliver' depends crucially on change and evolution at the level of the PHCT. This will require, amongst other things, a re-examination of roles, a breakdown of hierarchical structures, and new approaches to power sharing.

Within the model of the PHCT 'as we know it' lie some of the great strengths of British primary care, undoubtedly further strengthened by the NHS reforms. Its weaknesses, however, are also barriers to realising its true potential and rising to the challenges of the new agenda. Before examining some of these challenges – in other words looking at where we are now – it is worth considering how we got here in the first place.

How did we get here?

The *Oxford English Dictionary* offers one definition of a team as 'two or more beasts of burden harnessed together', and this image will appeal to many workers in primary care, certainly towards the end of a busy working week. In this sense the PHCT has been with us for a long time. Fry (1993) describes the original health team as the single-handed general practitioner working from home. He (usually) was assisted by his wife, who often combined the roles of receptionist, nurse and dispenser.

Since that time, the evolution of the PHCT as we know it today has paralleled that of primary care itself, taking place in fits and starts, piecemeal and *ad hoc* rather than strategic or planned. None the less, as Kuenssberg observes:

> It is impressive how development of the team took place unheralded, unstructured but the logical result of need and requirement, not something thought up by committees or legislators, though these were of course required to create a favourable environment.
>
> (Kuenssberg, 1991)

The introduction of reimbursement for ancillary staff in the mid-1960s (British Medical Association, 1965) saw the beginning of expansion, which was further fuelled by the 1974 reorganisation of the NHS, in which community nursing moved from local authority to health authority control. Increasing awareness of the scope of the task for primary care, set out in the Alma-Ata Declaration of 1978, and a succession of further social and legislative changes (for example, the 1990 NHS and Community Care Act) have reinforced the requirement for greater numbers of staff with a wider range of skills to meet the health needs of the community.

Milestones in the evolution of the PHCT have been documented in detail elsewhere (see, for example, Kuenssberg, 1991). However, it is evident that every major report on general practice and primary care has extolled the virtues of the team, from the Dawson Report in 1920 (Dawson, 1920) right through to the present (see, for example, Secretary of State for Health, 1996).

Collings, in his classic paper on the 'state of the art' of British general practice just after the inception of the NHS, argued the case for the creation, through resynthesis of all that is good in the traditional concept of family doctoring, of 'basic group-practice units'. He contends that 'in this modern age such a resynthesis implies teamwork between doctors, nurses, social workers and technicians, with the general practitioner as the co-ordinating agent of the team' (Collings, 1950). In 1981, the Harding Report (Standing Medical Advisory Committee and Standing Nursing and Midwifery Advisory Committee, 1981) went a step further and suggested that teamwork in primary care, especially between doctors and nurses, would produce better outcomes for patients.

Nevertheless, although the PHCT is widely advocated as the best means for delivering health care in the community, there are problems in realising this ambition. Many of these derive from the way in which primary care itself has evolved, and they include professional territorialism or 'tribalism' (Soothill *et al.*, 1995), different management structures, inequities in remuneration and status, and lack of common objectives, to name but a few. Neither is there consensus about what constitutes a team, or about the situations in which teams may, or may not be essential for optimal care. Furthermore, there are few useful outcome measures for teamwork (Jones, 1992). In fact, critical evidence to inform developments has been conspicuous by its absence. Instead, there has arisen 'a mythology of universal teamwork' (Stanley and Hatcher, 1992), in which the PHCT has become the panacea for all of the ills in the system.

Much of the published literature on teamwork in primary care has in the past been more rhetoric than evidence-based, the underlying assumption being that the PHCT is 'a good thing'. From Pinsent *et al.* in 1961 to Lambert in 1991, many and varied authors have offered passionate, eloquent and convincing arguments in favour of the PHCT, but little in the way of evidence of effectiveness and efficiency.

Exploring the mysteries of the primary health care team

None the less, various workers *have* attempted to explore the mysteries of PHCT function. Three examples will be given here. In 1974, Gilmore *et al.* described, from a nursing perspective, the essential features of effective teamworkers. They share a common purpose which guides their actions, each has a clear understanding of his or her own functions and roles, the team works by pooling knowledge, skills and resources, and all share a common responsibility for outcomes (Gilmore *et al.*, 1974). Gregson and her colleagues in Newcastle upon Tyne carried out a detailed study of the degree of collaboration between general practitioners, district nurses and health visitors in the mid-1980s, and highlighted the generally low level of working together that prevailed at that time. Among other things, they argued the case for both a shared physical base and shared patient records in order to facilitate better collaboration (Gregson *et al.*, 1991). Finally, Thomas approached primary care teamwork from an educational perspective, using a modification of a framework developed in psychoanalysis. She then applied the framework to both the analysis and the design of educational initiatives in primary care (Thomas, 1995).

These studies, which have approached teamwork from three quite different perspectives, remind us that diversity is one of the key features of primary care, certainly on a global scale (World Health Organization, 1978). Primary care must respond to people's needs, and these will vary from inner city to outer suburb, and from remote hamlet to market town. No single perspective is the 'right' one, and the challenge to those trying to promote teamwork in primary care (or to carry out research on it) is to try and reconcile the differences without sacrificing the dynamic tension that can itself produce creativity.

Despite the relative dearth of research on the development of the PHCT, there is a substantial body of evidence from other (non-health service) settings which shows that teamwork, underpinned by certain principles, can lead to increased effectiveness and efficiency. These principles, or pre-conditions, for effective team functioning include the following: having intrinsically interesting tasks to perform; individuals feeling that their contribution is important to the outcome; individual tasks that are meaningful and rewarding; individual contributions being reviewed, with feedback; and clear goals with regular feedback on performance (Guzzo and Shea, 1992).

Where are we now?

The 1980s and 1990s have seen dramatic changes in health care, most of which have major implications for the PHCT. Some of these changes, and the consequent challenges that they present, are considered below, and Pauline Pearson will return to some of these themes in the concluding chapter.

The purchaser–provider split

The introduction of the internal market and, with it, the 'purchaser–provider split', which is arguably one of the most profound changes of the NHS reforms, have increasingly shaped the pattern of health care provision in the UK in the 1990s. Within the legislation (Department of Health, 1990), general practice fundholding was created and, at the time of writing, over half the UK population are registered with a fundholding practice, a figure which is rising. The nature of fundholding has gradually evolved, and in its latest incarnations – so-called 'community fundholding' and 'total purchasing' – practices are able to purchase not only some or all hospital services for their patients, but also community services. An alternative purchasing strategy, namely locality commissioning, has evolved in parallel. This involves bringing together a group of practices in order to decide priorities for purchasing and to advise the health authority accordingly. Locality purchasing has been relatively successful in pilot schemes (Smith *et al.*, 1996), and is now being more widely implemented. Both models have implications for the way in which the PHCT functions. For instance, total purchasing, in allowing fund-holders to purchase community nursing services, for the first time gives doctors the right to decide what health visitors and district nurses should be doing.

Community care

Another major strand of the NHS reforms is the NHS and Community Care Act (Department of Health, 1990), which set in train a number of changes in the way in which health and social care was provided to vulnerable groups, such as the elderly or those with mental health problems. The major changes were a shift towards an internal market for social care, with the development on the one hand of the 'care manager' holding the budget for social care for a given group, and on the other hand the 'care provider' (social worker, district nurse, home carer, etc.), together with an increasing emphasis on the role of independent (voluntary or private sector) provision, and encouragement for joint purchasing between health and social care agencies. These changes have considerable implications for the PHCT. Attempts to decide what is health care and what is social care, who should be providing that care, where and when, inevitably beg questions about membership of the PHCT and roles within it. Working across sector boundaries as well as professional boundaries adds new dimensions to the problems of 'tribalism' (Soothill *et al.*, 1995).

Needs assessment

This is an area of development which has emerged as important in the wake of the major policy and legislative changes that took place during the last decade. Purchasing, community care, and Health of the Nation (Department of Health, 1991) are three areas in which an assessment of the needs of the population served by the PHCT is clearly necessary in order to permit rational decisions about health care priorities and provision. Some members of the PHCT may be better able to develop a leading role in this area, for instance health visitors, who have traditionally seen health needs assessment as one of their key roles.

Evidence-based practice

Against the background of a rising demand for, and expectations of, health care within limited resources, together with increasing awareness of variations in quality of care, there is now increasing acceptance of the need to ensure clinical effectiveness through a variety of means, including protocols and guidelines, clinical audit, and continuous quality improvement. Evidence-based practice is advocated as the best framework for achieving the goal of clinical effectiveness, and is defined as 'the conscientious, explicit and judicious use of current best evidence in making decisions about the care of individual patients. The practice of evidence-based healthcare means integrating individual clinical expertise with the best available, external clinical evidence from systematic research' (Sackett *et al.*, 1996). Clearly this is not a uniprofessional issue, since changes in the practice of any single professional group within a team will impinge on the work of others. The challenge of introducing evidence-based practice into the day-to-day working of the PHCT is considerable, and a multifaceted approach will certainly be needed (Jones *et al.*, 1996).

The changing role of the 'patient'

One of the major changes in the past 20 years has been the emergence of the 'consumer' in health care, not least in primary care. It is stating the obvious to say that the main goal of health care should be improvement in the health status of individuals and populations, and all changes in policy, philosophy and practice have implications for 'the patient'. Yet most models of the PHCT see the team as an organisation doing something to or for the patient. Efforts to incorporate the patient's perspective have been patchy and have achieved only modest success (with respect to patient participation groups see, for example, Pietroni and Chase, 1993). The issues have been eloquently debated by Williamson, who argues that 'the real challenge for the future' is moving from paternalism to partnership, whilst ensuring that respect for the unique value of the individual – one of the traditional strengths of the doctor–patient relationship in general practice – is embedded at the heart of multidisciplinary teamwork in primary care (Williamson, 1996).

Reconstructing general practice

General practice as a profession has undergone major change in the past decade, much of it imposed or reactive in nature, resulting in a sense of powerlessness, increased managerial control, loss of independence, and general demoralisation. This has contributed to increasing numbers of early retirements from general practice and a serious recruitment crisis. Further-more, whereas the rhetoric of the 'primary care-led NHS' was about bringing service delivery and decisions concerning priorities as close as possible to the patient (National Health Service Executive, 1994), this has often been experienced at the 'coalface' as a strategic shift of care unsupported by evidence of efficacy, implemented without adequate consultation, and not matched by a shift of resources. It is also evident that policy-makers and managers wish to exploit the cost-effectiveness of British primary care whilst not fully understanding 'the nature of the subtle transactions that make that cost-effectiveness possible' (Fugelli and Heath, 1996). General practice has been forced to re-examine the very nature of the discipline in an attempt to define its content, set boundaries and regain some control over its destiny. Key strands in this process have included the following: reiterating the enduring strengths of general practice, namely continuity, clinical generalism, the gatekeeper function, and multi-disciplinary teamworking (Royal College of General Practitioners, 1996); defining 'core' and 'non-core' services (General Medical Services

Committee, 1996); exploring new ways of extending and delivering primary care, e.g. through resource centres or polyclinics and taking stock of the options for purchasing and commissioning (Gordon and Hadley, 1996); and finally revisiting some of the great shibboleths of general practice, such as the 24-hour commitment and out-of-hours arrangements.

Many of these themes are reflected in the latest policy documents (for example, *Choice and Opportunity. Primary Care: The Future*). In the new climate of flexibility and diversity, developments such as different contractual options for general practitioners, e.g. a salaried service for inner-city general practice or practice-based contracts, and extending the roles and responsibilities of other health professionals, e.g. nurses, through the evolution of the nurse practitioner and an extension of nurse prescribing, all have profound implications for the way in which the PHCT functions.

In the context of these changes it is more important than ever that we explore the complexities of the PHCT, in particular in order to deepen our understanding of the crucial issue of how best to promote effective team functioning – the focus of the present book. In this book we have brought together the work of a number of individuals, a truly multidisciplinary group, who offer a variety of perspectives on this issue. We also make some suggestions about a future agenda for research into the PHCT.

Chapter 2 sets primary health care teams within their wider context. West and Poulton outline some of the teamwork literature from organisational psychology, and challenge assumptions such as the view that the group is greater than the sum of its parts. They then describe findings from a study of team effectiveness which showed primary health care teams consistently falling behind the other teams studied. They conclude by indicating some areas for improvement of team effectiveness in primary care, based on their research findings.

Chapter 3 explores the detailed composition of primary care teams. It briefly examines the historical development of UK general practice and primary care, before describing changes in the shape of practice teams following the introduction of the 1990 GP contract. Usherwood and his colleagues introduce the notion of a 'typical practice team' in their discussion of study data. They conclude by examining the factors that are likely to affect the future composition of primary health care teams.

Chapter 4 shifts focus in order to examine the everyday work of informal teams in community settings. Edward describes the complex nature of day-to-day interactions, and the ways in which professionals negotiate their patterns of work. She highlights the need for flexibility, accessibility and valuing the contributions of others in order to produce effective team-working.

Chapter 5 looks at a large-scale practical example of work to promote team development in primary care. Bryar describes the Teamcare Valleys initiative in South Wales, which was set up with central government funding to encourage improved teamwork and develop primary care. In describing this innovative, multifaceted approach, she draws examples from each of the four main programme areas, and highlights key outcome areas.

In Chapter 6, Gooding outlines the philosophy and practice of one of the best known programmes of team development, namely that run by the Health Education Authority, in which 10 per cent of practices in England and Wales participated. She describes the changes which have occurred since its beginnings in 1987, outlines the results of evaluation, and discusses plans for future development.

Chapter 7 takes us to the other end of the scale, centring on the use of a practice manifesto to set out interdisciplinary aims and objectives in one primary health care team. Freake and van Zwanenberg examine how this works in practice, and explore the potential of this type of approach as a means of drawing together a multidisciplinary team, as well as how manifestos and patient charters relate to one another.

Chapter 8 again involves examination of a local intervention. Spencer and Southern describe a project working with five practices in the North East to explore and promote team function, and then build up a framework for multi-disciplinary audit. They conclude that, although not all of the teams involved completed the task set, team functioning was facilitated, and a climate was created in which multidisciplinary audit was more likely to occur.

Audit is the means by which practitioners can examine the impact of their work. In Chapter 9, Baker and Hearnshaw consider further the evidence with regard to multidisciplinary audit in primary health care teams and its impact on patient care. They review one model for the management of audit by a primary health care team, and discuss the applicability of commercial models of quality improvement. They go on to examine the effect of focused facilitation on the implementation of multidisciplinary audit, indicating the potential of this approach. However, they conclude that there remains insufficient evidence to justify the investment of scarce resources for intro-ducing multidisciplinary audit more widely, and suggest that further research must be undertaken in this area.

Chapter 10 describes three studies in which aspects of team function were evaluated. Methodological issues arising from these are discussed, and the questions addressed include sampling and variability, data col-lection options and intentions, time, resourcing, ownership and impact of evaluation.

Chapter 11 presents material from a large-scale study designed to define and measure effectiveness for primary health care teams. Poulton and West describe the development of an empirical framework for use in assessing effectiveness, and outline the ways in which this was operationalised by them. They explore the measurement of team structures and processes, and the development of measures of output. They indicate that the possession of clear, shared objectives is the largest single predictor of effectiveness for primary health care teams.

In Chapter 12, Pearson and Spencer look more globally at outcome measures for teamwork in primary care. They sketch out the priorities found in a Delphi study, and analyse these priorities according to the respondents' experience of primary care. Some differences are identified between those respondents who had worked in primary care, and those who had not, and the implications of these findings are discussed.

Chapter 13 is the first of two chapters which explore the use of an action research approach in work on team development. Thomas and Graver outline the genesis of the Liverpool intervention to promote teamwork in general practice, and the development of a framework for evaluation. The Liverpool intervention was built up in three stages to promote inter-disciplinary working across the city. Thomas and Graver suggest that individual, service, organisational and contextual changes must all be explored in order to obtain a clear picture of the impact of a complex intervention.

In Chapter 14, Hudson and Bennett take up the theme of action research and describe its use in two quite different projects in individual practices on Tayside. The first project explored stress within a primary health care team, and the second looked at the introduction of a 'patient services manager' within a team. Issues addressed in the discussion include the problems which arise from the short-term reactive approach to much development work in primary care, the importance of a flexible, participative approach to project-based work of this type, and the need to look carefully at the role of the researcher in relation to the various stakeholders.

Finally, in Chapter 15, Pearson reviews some of the current determinants of change in primary health care. She links these to their likely impact on teamwork in primary care, and develops a 'vision' for the future. In conclusion, she discusses some of the research agendas which may result.

Editors' summary

In this chapter, Spencer has provided a brief overview of the evolution of the idea of the primary health care team, together with an insight into some of the developments currently taking place. In the era of the 'primary care-led NHS' he has pointed out some of the exciting challenges and opportunities which lie ahead. All of these have major implications for teamwork in primary health care. Finally, he has briefly summarised the chapters which follow, in order to give a flavour of what is to come.

References

British Medical Association (1965) A charter for the family doctor service. *British Medical Journal Supplement* 1, 89–91.

Collings JS (1950) General practice in England today: a reconnaissance. *Lancet* 1, 555–85.

Dawson B (1920) *Report on the Future Provision of Medical and Allied Services*. Cm 693. HMSO, London.

Department of Health (1990) *NHS and Community Care Act 1990*. HMSO, London.

Department of Health (1991) *The Health of the Nation*. HMSO, London.

Fry J (1993) *General Practice: The Facts*. Radcliffe Medical Press, Oxford.

Fugelli P and Heath I (1996) The nature of general practice. Yes to traditional values must mean no to fundholding and managerial ambition. *British Medical Journal* 312, 456–7.

General Medical Services Committee (1996) *Core Services: Taking the Initiative*. British Medical Association, London.

Gilmore M, Bruce N and Hunt M (1974) *The Work of the Nursing Team in General Practice*. Council for the Education and Training of Health Visitors, London.

Gordon P and Hadley J (eds) (1996) *Extending Primary Care*. Radcliffe Medical Press, Oxford.

Gregson BA, Cartlidge A and Bond J (1991) *Interprofessional Collaboration in Primary Health Care Organizations. Occasional Paper 52*. Royal College of General Practitioners, London.

Guzzo RA and Shea GP (1992) Group performance and intergroup relations in organizations. In Dunnette D and Hough LM (eds) *Handbook of Industrial and Organizational Psychology*, pp. 269–313. Counselling Psychologists Press, Palo Alto.

Jarman B and Cumberlege J (1987) Developing primary health care. *British Medical Journal* 294, 1005–8.

Jones K, Wilson A, Russell I *et al.* (1996) Evidence-based practice in primary care. *British Journal of Community Health Nursing* 1, 276–80.

Jones RVH (1992) Teamwork in primary care: how much do we know about it? *Journal of Interprofessional Care* 6, 25–30.

Kuenssberg EV (1991) The team in primary care (1930–1990). In *Royal College of General Practitioners Members' Reference Book*, pp. 433–8. Sabrecrown Publishers, London.

Lambert D (1991) Developing primary health care teams. *Primary Health Care Management* 12, 2–3.

NHS Executive (1994) *Developing NHS Purchasing and GP Fundholding: Towards a Primary Care-Led NHS*. Department of Health, Leeds.

Pietroni P and Chase HD (1993) Partners or partisans? Patient participation at Marylebone Health Centre. *British Journal of General Practice* 43, 341–4.

Pinsent R, Pike L, Morgan R *et al.* (1961) The health visitor in a general practice. *British Medical Journal Supplement* 1, 123–7.

Royal College of General Practitioners (1996) *The Nature of General Medical Practice. Report from General Practice 27*. Royal College of General Practitioners, London.

Sackett DL, Rosenberg WM, Gray JA, Haynes RB and Richardson WS (1996) Evidence-based medicine: what it is and what it isn't. *British Medical Journal* 312, 71–2.

Secretary of State for Health (1996) *Primary Care: Delivering the Future*. HMSO, London.

Smith R, Butler F and Powell M (eds) (1996) *Total Purchasing. A Model for Locality Commissioning*. Radcliffe Medical Press, Oxford.

Soothill K, Mackay L and Webb C (1995) *Intraprofessional Relations in Health Care.* Edward Arnold, London.

Standing Medical Advisory Committee and Standing Nursing and Midwifery Advisory Committee (1981) *The Primary Health Care Team: Report of a Joint Working Group (Harding Committee).* HMSO, London.

Stanley I and Hatcher P (1992) The PHCT: realising the myth. *Good Practice,* April 1992, 17–19.

Thomas M (1995) Learning to be a better team-player: initiatives in continuing education in primary health care. In Soothill K, Mackay L and Webb C (eds) *Interprofessional Relations in Health Care,* pp. 194–214. Edward Arnold, London.

Waine C (1992) The primary care team. *British Journal of General Practice* 42, 498–9.

Williamson V (1996) Personal care and teamwork in primary care: the patient's perspective. *Journal of Interprofessional Care* 9, 101–6.

World Health Organization (1978) *Alma-Ata 1978. Primary Health Care: Report of the International Conference.* World Health Organization, Geneva.

2

Primary health care teams: in a league of their own

Michael West and Brenda Poulton

Introduction

In this chapter we describe the nature of work groups or teams and examine the reasons for their use in organisations, and in primary health care in particular. The very real problems and difficulties of working in teams are described, and mechanisms for overcoming them are suggested. In this context, the functioning of primary health care teams is examined, and ways of improving primary health care team effectiveness are outlined.

What is a work group or team?

Formal work groups are those which have an identity and set of functions derived from and contributing to the achievement of organisational objectives. Such groups occur in many different forms. They include project groups (e.g. a research and development group exploring new ways of putting plastic cabling on to wheels), multidisciplinary groups (e.g. a nurse, physiotherapist and counsellor collaborating to plan treatment for victims of road traffic accidents), cross-functional groups (e.g. representatives from marketing, production, sales and research and development), semi-autonomous work groups who are largely responsible for their own work planning and processes, quality improvement groups (e.g. a group attempting to reduce the level of customer complaints), functional groups (e.g. surgical groups and airline flight crews) and, of course, primary health care teams (Hackman, 1990).

What characterises formal groups or teams? (The terms 'group' and 'team' will be used interchangeably in this chapter.) First, members of a group have shared objectives with regard to their work. They depend on and must interact with one another in order to achieve those objectives. Group members have more or less well-defined roles, some of which are differentiated from each other (e.g. in the primary health care team, doctors, nurses and receptionists), and they have an organisational identity as a work group with a defined organisational function (e.g. a public relations group for a pharmaceutical company), i.e. they perceive themselves, and others in the organisation see them, as a defined and bounded group. Finally, they are not so large that they would be defined more appropriately as an organisation with an internal structure of vertical and horizontal relationships, characterised by sub-groups. In practice, this is likely to mean that the work group will have less than about 20 members, although clearly there would be exceptions to this (Goodman *et al.*, 1986; Guzzo and Shea, 1992; West, 1996).

Why do we organise work in groups?

Work groups are formed because of a belief that, in some circumstances, having people work on shared goals interdependently will lead to synergy – the aggregate of individuals' performances will be exceeded by the work group's performance. Furthermore, it is believed that, by bringing together diverse skills and integrating them, the achievement of organisational goals may be more successful. For example, the skills of nurses, administrators and doctors in a primary health care group will better meet the health needs of the local population if they are integrated and combined, rather than distributed and perhaps competing. Moreover, groups enable organisations to maintain memories. If one person leaves the group, important information is not necessarily lost, but continues to be maintained in the group memory. A similar argument can be applied to the experience of the group. Knowledge and skills of functioning are retained even if one member is absent, or leaves the group.

As organisations have grown in size and become structurally more complex, the need for groups of people to work together in co-ordinated ways in order to achieve objectives that contribute to the overall aims of the organisation has become increasingly clear. Similarly, technology has changed within the last 50 years, with the burgeoning of information technology. Such complexity requires more intricate structures or groupings of people in response.

Clearly, work groups are not appropriate for every task or function within an organisation, but there is evidence that the introduction of group goals leads to better performance and productivity in a variety of work settings. Examples cited in a review of more than 30 studies of group goals and group performance (Weldon and Weingart, 1993) include the following: loading trucks; performing work safely; harvesting and hauling timber; opening mail; operating spinning machines; running a restaurant; processing insurance appraisals; and raising money for voluntary organisations. Specific, difficult goals have been found to improve the performance of groups much more than vague 'do your best' or easily attainable goals. When group members feel an attachment to the goal and feel strongly that the group should reach that goal (a situation known as 'goal commitment'), not surprisingly goal attainment is more likely. Weldon and Weingart (1993) have suggested a number of factors which may determine the commitment of group members to a group goal. These include the following: the attractiveness of goal attainment (e.g. the group goal being compatible with group members' personal goals); the fact that membership of the group may lead to satisfaction of individual desires (perhaps simply by being part of a successful or attractive group); having a charismatic group leader; group members' expectations that the group can successfully complete its task; competing demands that will reduce the likelihood of goal attainment (e.g. the deleterious effects of conflicts between seeking to provide excellent patient care in hospitals, demands to reduce health care costs, and demands to do work narrowly defined according to professional identity – 'that's nurses' work, not doctors''); goal commitment of others in the group; and goal difficulty (if the group goal is perceived to be too difficult to attain, the level of commitment may be reduced).

Weldon and Weingart have also described the importance of planning in groups for achieving group goals, and suggest that group members are characteristically slow to respond to changes in their tasks or in their environments that make their strategies ineffective or their goals obsolete. They propose five ways of supporting group work.

- Goals should be set for all dimensions of performance that contribute to the overall effectiveness of the group.
- Feedback should be provided on the group's progress towards its goal.
- The physical environment of the group should remove barriers to effective interaction (e.g. being based in different health centres).
- Group members should be encouraged to plan carefully how their contributions can be identified and co-ordinated to achieve the group goal.
- Group members should be helped to manage failure, which can damage the subsequent effectiveness of the group.

Problems of working in groups

There is a good deal of research evidence which suggests that, regardless of goals, in some circumstances groups may perform less effectively than individuals working alone, and that certain aspects of group processes can interfere with the attempts of groups to perform optimally in work settings.

Early this century, a French agricultural engineer attempted to discover whether individuals working alone were more effective than those working in groups (Ringelmann, 1913). He instructed agricultural students to pull on a rope attached to a dynamometer, and he measured the amount of pull. Working alone, the average student could pull a weight of around 85 kilograms. Ringelmann then assigned the students to groups of seven, for which the average pull was 450 kilograms. The groups were pulling only 75 per cent as hard as the aggregated effort of seven individuals.

Further research has involved groups solving conceptual problems, e.g. how to transport sheep and hungry wolves safely across a river in a boat. Although groups took longer than individuals, they achieved more correct solutions. Other tasks involved '20 questions' games. Here a particular object is selected but not identified, and players have to guess the name of the object by asking up to 20 questions, to which they are given only a 'yes' or 'no' answer. Groups have been found to be slightly more effective than individuals in arriving at correct solutions within their 20 questions, but they tend to be less efficient with regard to time use. Individuals took, on average, 5 minutes to reach the correct solution. Groups of two took 7 person-minutes (i.e. 3.5 minutes in real time) and groups of four required 12 person-minutes (3 minutes in real time). There were no differences between groups of two and four people with regard to the probability of a correct answer (see Brown, 1988, for a review of these studies).

Group functioning can therefore sometimes be less effective than the aggregate of individual efforts. The term 'process losses' is used to refer to the various group processes which hinder effective group functioning (Steiner, 1972). But what are these process losses? One phenomenon identified by social psychologists is 'social loafing'. Individuals work less hard when their efforts are combined with and masked by those of others than when they are individually accountable (Latané *et al.*, 1979). The social loafing problem challenges the assumption of group 'synergy', that teams are always more effective than the sum of the contributions of their individual members. Are problems of group working therefore confined simply to this relative lack of effort among group members? Studies of group decision-making suggest that there are other forms of process loss which hinder effective group functioning in very different ways.

One of the most important reasons why people work in groups is so that they can use their diverse knowledge, skills and experiences to contribute to achievement of the best possible decisions. In determining where and how to drill for oil, the knowledge of geologists, engineers and chemists needs to be co-ordinated. Indeed, a principal assumption underlying the structuring of organisational activities into work groups is that groups will make better decisions than individual members working alone. However, research clearly indicates that while groups make decisions of a better quality than the average quality of decisions made by individual members (rated by experts external to the group), work groups consistently fall short of the quality of decisions made by their most capable individual members (Rogelberg *et al.*, 1992). Organisational and social psychologists have therefore attempted to identify the processes which impede effective group decision-making. The following issues have been identified.

Personality factors such as shyness can cause some group members to hesitate in offering their opinions and knowledge assertively, so that they thereby fail to contribute fully to the group's store of knowledge. Egocentricity may lead others to be unwilling to consider opinions contrary to their own. Group members are also subject to social conformity effects, causing them to withhold opinions and information contrary to the majority view, especially if that is an organisationally dominant view (Brown, 1988). Members of work groups may lack communication skills and so be unable to present their views and knowledge successfully. There may be domination by particular individuals who take up disproportionate 'air time', or who argue so vigorously with the opinions of others that their own views prevail. It is noteworthy that 'air time' and expertise are correlated in high-performing groups and uncorrelated in groups that perform poorly (Rogelberg *et al.*, 1992). Status, gender and hierarchy effects (e.g. male GPs vs. female nurses) can also cause some members' contributions to be valued and attended to disproportionately. When the senior GP partner is present in a meeting, his (usually) or her views are likely to have a considerable influence on the outcome.

'Risky shift', or group polarisation, is the tendency of work groups to make more extreme decisions than the average of individual members' decisions. Group decisions tend to be either more risky or more conservative than the average of individual members' opinions or decisions. When individuals discover the position of others, they tend to move along the scale of opinion partly because of a 'majority rule' influence – the largest sub-group tends to determine the group decision. Moreover, a process of social comparison may take place, whereby information about a socially preferred way of behaving leads to polarisation. When we compare ourselves with those immediately around us in the organisation, we tend to locate our position closer to theirs, rather than retaining the integrity of our initial position. Within organisations, the dangers of polarisation are greatest when the group has just been formed, or when the group is confronted with an unusual situation (often a crisis). Thus shifts in the extremity of decisions affecting the competitive strategy of an organisation can occur simply as a result of group processes, rather than for rational or well-judged reasons (Myers and Lamm, 1976).

The 'social loafing' effect (see above) can extend to information-seeking and decision-making. Individuals may put less effort into achieving high-quality decisions in meetings, as a result of their perception that their contribution will be hidden in overall group performance. Diffusion of responsibility can also inhibit individuals from taking responsibility for action when working with others. People often assume that responsibility will be shouldered by others who are present in a situation requiring action (Darley and Latané, 1968). In organisational settings, individuals may fail to act in a crisis involving the functioning of expensive technology, judging that others in their team are taking responsibility for making the necessary decisions. Consequently, the overall quality of group decisions can be threatened.

The study of 'brainstorming' groups has regularly shown that the quantity, and often quality, of ideas produced by individuals working separately consistently exceed those of ideas produced by a group working together (Diehl and Stroebe, 1987). Early studies comparing the effectiveness of brainstorming individually or in groups involved creating 'statisticised' and 'real' groups. Statisticised groups consisted of five individuals, working alone in separate rooms, who were given a 5-minute period in which to generate ideas about uses for an object. Their results were then aggregated, and any redundancies due to repetition of ideas by different individuals were removed. Real groups of five individuals worked together for 5 minutes, generating as many ideas as possible and withholding criticism. The statisticised groups were found to produce an average of 68 ideas, while the real groups produced an average of only 37 ideas. In over 20 studies this finding has almost always been confirmed. Individuals working alone produce more ideas, of at least as high a quality when they are aggregated, than groups working together. Research by social psychologists clearly indicates that this counter-intuitive finding is due to a 'production-blocking' effect (Diehl and Stroebe, 1987). When people are speaking in brainstorming groups, others are not able to speak and so (temporarily) cannot put ideas forward. Moreover, because they may be holding ideas in their memories, waiting for a chance to speak, their ability to produce more ideas is impaired. Individuals are thus inhibited by the competing verbalisations of others from both thinking of new ideas and presenting them aloud to the group.

Another process which occurs during group decision-making is 'satisficing' or making decisions immediately acceptable to the group, rather than the best possible decisions (Cyert and March, 1963). Video and audiotape recordings of group decision-making processes show that groups often identify the first minimally acceptable solution or decision, and then spend time searching for reasons to accept that decision and reject other possible options. They tend not to generate a range of alternatives before selecting, on a rational basis, the most suitable option. Finally, Janis (1982), in his studies of government policy decisions and fiascos, suggested a group syndrome which he called 'groupthink', whereby cohesive groups may err in their decision-making, as a result of being more concerned with achieving agreement than with the quality of group decision-making (a process we shall discuss in more detail later). This can be especially threatening to organisational functioning where different departments see themselves as competing with one another, promoting 'in-group' favouritism and therefore a greater likelihood of groupthink.

Group decision-making is therefore more complex and problematic than is commonly perceived within organisational settings. Recently, researchers have begun to identify ways to overcome some of these deficiencies. For example, research on 'groupthink' suggests both that the phenomenon is most likely to occur in groups where a manager is particularly dominant, and that cohesiveness *per se* is not a crucial factor (McCauley, 1989). This suggests that managers (or GPs) could be trained to be facilitative, seeking the contributions of individual members before offering their own perceptions (Field and West, 1995). Given the problems confronting those seeking to work effectively in groups, what evidence is there of the effectiveness of primary health care teams compared to others?

How effective are primary health care teams?

In one study (West and Poulton, 1996), we compared primary health care teams with other multidisciplinary teams with regard to four fundamental dimensions of team functioning:

- clarity of, and team member commitment to, team objectives;
- levels of participation within the teams (information sharing, frequency of team member interaction, and extent of team member influence over decision-making);
- task orientation or commitment to excellence;
- support for innovation.

We shall describe each of the four elements of team functioning in further detail below.

Objectives

Work groups with clearly defined objectives are more likely to be effective and to develop new goal-appropriate methods of working, because their efforts have focus and direction.

Participation

Wall and Lischeron (1977) describe participation as having three central components. Interaction involves '... two parties attempting to reach agreement through working together rather than through recourse to a balance of power based upon the exercise of sanctions'. Information sharing, they say, is also central to participation since '... interaction between the two parties undertaken with the ultimate aim of reaching agreement over a decision, requires and results in an exchange of information and increased intercommunication'. Finally, they argue, participation may be said to increase 'to the extent that the influence of two or more parties in a decision-making process approaches an equal balance'.

Task orientation

A shared concern about excellence of quality of task performance in relation to shared vision or outcomes, characterised by evaluations, modifications, control systems and critical appraisals, is the third component. Within teams this is evidenced by emphasis on individual and team accountability, control systems for evaluating and modifying performance, critical approaches to quality of task performance, intra-team advice, feedback and co-operation, mutual monitoring, appraisal of performance and ideas, clear outcome criteria, exploration of opposing opinions, and a concern to maximise quality of task performance.

Support for innovation

The fourth and final component is support for innovation, or the expectation and approval of, and practical support for, attempts to introduce new and improved ways of performing tasks in the work environment. At the organisational level such norms may be explicit in the socialisation practices for incumbents or implicit in the culture of the organisation. Within groups, new ideas may be characteristically rejected or ignored, or find both verbal and practical support.

Within a work group characterised by support for innovation, all members of a primary health care team might be encouraged to contribute to discussions and decision-making about important aspects of the team's work. At the same time, the team's characteristic interpersonal processes would be non-judgemental and supportive of the individual offering contributions and suggestions, and characterised by socio-emotional cohesiveness.

The study

Data on these dimensions of team functioning were collected from 528 members of 68 primary health care teams located throughout the UK. These included 106 general practitioners, 63 health visitors, 44 district nurses, 56 practice nurses, 118 receptionists, 42 practice managers and 99 others (e.g. midwives, counsellors, community psychiatric nurses). The teams were nominated for the most part by Local Organising Teams involved in facilitating Health Education Authority team workshops (see Chapter 6). Data were also obtained from the following four samples of multi-disciplinary teams: 200 members of 24 oil company management teams; 155 members of 27 NHS hospital top management teams; 120 members of 20 community mental health teams; and 360 members of 40 social services teams. Further details of these samples and the methods of data collection can be found in Anderson and West (1994). All teams included in the sample responded to a questionnaire survey and were only included if four members or 40 per cent of members of the team responded (whichever was the larger figure).

The instrument used to measure the four elements of team functioning – objectives, participation, task orientation, and support for innovation – was the Team Climate Inventory. This inventory has been validated by comparing team member responses with analyses of audio tapes of interaction processes in team meetings, and it shows high criterion, content and face validity (see Anderson and West, 1994). Its reliability on all four scales has also been shown to be high. In addition, two measures of mutual role understanding within the teams were included in the questionnaire, together with primary health care team members' perceptions of whether other members made appropriate use of their skills. As well as questionnaire administration, intensive case studies of primary health care team work were conducted on 10 teams in order to gain a more qualitative appreciation of the challenges and difficulties faced by the different professional groups in attempting to co-ordinate their work effectively.

Analyses of the data revealed considerable variation in the size of primary health care teams, ranging from the smallest with seven members up to the largest with 37 members (see also Chapter 3). The average size of primary health care teams in the study was 18 members. Given that most organisational behaviourists view the maximum effective team size as being between 8 and 12 members, this finding suggests that some of the difficulties of primary health care teams may derive from the assumption that groups of 20–40 individuals can be managed as work teams (see, for example, Guzzo and Shea, 1992). Large primary health care teams should correctly be considered as small organisations rather than as teams.

The scores across the five samples of work groups (primary health care teams, NHS management teams, community mental health teams, oil company management teams and social services teams) were compared using standard analyses of variance. We found significant differences between primary health care teams and the other work groups on all four dimensions (West and Poulton, 1997). On every scale but one (task orientation), primary health care teams scored lowest of the five samples. Moreover, primary health care teams reported significantly lower levels of participation than teams in each of the other samples, significantly lower levels of support for innovation than those reported by NHS management teams and community mental health teams, significantly less clarity of and commitment to objectives than any of the other four samples, and significantly lower levels of task orientation than community mental health teams and social services teams.

How can effectiveness in primary health care teamwork be improved?

There are two fundamental dimensions of team functioning, namely the task that the team is required to carry out, and the social factors which influence how members experience the team as a social unit. The basic reason for the creation of teams in work organisations is the expectation that they will carry out tasks more effectively than individuals and so further organisational objectives overall. Consideration of the content of the task, and the strategies and processes employed by team members to perform that task, is important for understanding how to work in teams. At the same time, teams are composed of people who have a variety of emotional, social and other human needs which the team as a whole can either help to meet or frustrate.

In order to function effectively, team members must actively focus upon their objectives, regularly reviewing ways of achieving them and the team's methods of working. At the same time, in order to promote the well-being of its members, the team must reflect upon the ways in which it provides support to members, how conflicts are resolved, and the overall social climate of the team – or its 'social reflexivity'. The purpose of these review processes should be to provide active steps to change the team's objectives, ways of working or social functioning, in order to promote effectiveness (for an extended discussion of those issues, see West, 1996).

What does 'team effectiveness' actually mean? It can be seen as having three main components:

- *task effectiveness* is the extent to which the team is successful in achieving its task-related objectives;
- *mental health* refers to the well-being, growth and development of team members;
- *team viability* is the probability that members of a team will continue to work together and function effectively as a team.

These two aspects of team functioning, i.e. task and social reflexivity, have a direct impact upon the three principal outcomes of team functioning, namely task effectiveness, team members' mental health, and team viability.

In what other ways can teams at work overcome some of the problems which have been identified so far, such as social loafing? Although the research described has not been encouraging with regard to the superiority of team work over individual work, nevertheless some very clear guidelines can be offered for increasing group effectiveness.

Groups should have intrinsically interesting tasks to perform

A good deal of research evidence indicates that people will work harder if the tasks they are asked to perform are intrinsically interesting, motivating, challenging and enjoyable. Where teams have an inherently interesting task to perform there is generally strong commitment, a higher level of motivation and more co-operative working. This therefore calls for very careful design of the objectives and tasks of work.

In many companies influenced by Japanese management practices, individuals work in relatively autonomous self-managing teams, redesigning work themselves to make tasks more meaningful and to improve quality of performance. Teams should be given tasks which are intrinsically interesting, but should also be given considerable autonomy in modifying task objectives to ensure that the team's goals help to maintain overall motivation. Clearly, the work of primary health care teams – promoting the health and well-being of the local population – is intrinsically motivating and likely to be seen as highly valued socially.

Individuals should feel that they are important to the fate of the group

Social loafing effects are most likely to occur when people believe that their contributions to the group are dispensable. For example, in primary health care teams, we have found that some members feel their work is not highly valued. Health visitors and receptionists are particularly likely to feel this way. One way in which individuals can begin to feel that their work is important to the fate of the group is through the use of techniques of *role clarification* and *negotiation*. By careful exploration of the roles of each team member, together with the identification of team and individual objectives, team members can see and demonstrate more clearly to other team members the importance of their work to the overall success of the team.

Individuals should have intrinsically interesting tasks to perform

Individual tasks should also be meaningful and inherently rewarding. Just as it is important for a group to have an intrinsically interesting task to perform, so too individuals will work harder and be more committed and creative if the tasks they are performing are engaging and challenging. For example, a researcher who is sitting in on team meetings and observing team processes is more motivated and has a more creative attitude towards the task than a researcher who is required to input the data from questionnaires on to a computer. Within primary health care teams, the diversity and responsibility of individual roles are generally very high, compared to (for example) jobs in manufacturing or heavy industries.

Individual contributions should be indispensable, unique and evaluated against a standard

Research on social loafing indicates that the effect is considerably reduced where people perceive their work to be indispensable to the performance of the team as a whole. It is equally important, however, that individual work should be subject to evaluation. People have to feel not only that their work is indispensable, but also that their performance is *visible* to other members of the team. In laboratory settings, where team members know that the products of their performance will be observed by other members of the team, they are much more likely to maintain effort to the level which they would achieve normally in individual performance. For example, when individuals are told that each team member's shouting will be measured in order to assess their individual contribution to the overall loudness of the team, the classic social loafing effect does not occur. Therefore, it is important within team settings for each team member to feel that his or her performance will be evaluated against a standard within the group, at the end of some specified period of team performance. For a general practitioner this might be measured by such factors as the number of surgery patients seen, the quality of clinical interactions with patients, patient satisfaction with the general practitioner, the number of home visits completed, the quality of clinical interactions during home visits, prescribing practices, and the quantity and quality of communications with other team members. In practice, we have found that *meaningful* performance evaluation and feedback for members of primary health care teams are largely non-existent. This is a major failure of performance management in this field.

There should be clear team goals with in-built performance feedback

For the same reasons that it is important for individuals to have clear goals and performance feedback, so too it is important for the team as a whole to have clear group goals with performance feedback. Research evidence shows very consistently that, where people are set clear targets, their performance is generally improved. However, goals can only function as a motivator of team performance if accurate performance feedback is available. For example, in the case of primary health care teams there should be performance feedback at least annually on all or some of the following indices (West, 1994):

- patient satisfaction with the quality of care given;
- the effectiveness of innovations and changes introduced by the team;
- the quality of clinical care given by the team;
- improvement in community health;
- the effectiveness with which team members have achieved their own objectives as a team;
- the quality of the team climate and how well team members feel they have worked together;
- the quality of intra-team communication;
- the quality of relationships with other agencies, such as social services, local authorities and hospitals;

- the financial effectiveness of the practice;
- the efficiency of the practice in reducing patient waiting times;
- improvement in patient access to health care and health promotion.

The more precise the indicators of team performance, the more likely a team is to improve its performance and inhibit the effects of social loafing. This is probably the single most important criterion for effective team functioning. However, it is in this area that primary health care team functioning, in our experience, presents the most difficulties. This failure to derive clear shared objectives from identified health needs in the local population, and then to evaluate progress towards achieving them, represents a fundamental threat to primary health care team effectiveness. In our view it derives from the structural difficulties created by diverse management structures in primary care (different management lines for health visitors, midwives, district nurses, practice nurses, GPs, practice managers and receptionists). Crucially, too, it is – in our view – a result of the anomalous status of GPs as independent contractors in teams of professionals who do not share that status or reward structure. This is a major impediment to the development of clear, shared, team-level objectives.

Conclusions

In this chapter we have offered three important and somewhat neglected perspectives in researchers' and practitioners' considerations about effective teamwork in primary health care. First, there is a need to recognise and draw upon the wealth of literature in organisational psychology and management which describes accumulated knowledge about teamwork more generally. Secondly, we have illustrated the apparent comparative weakness of teamwork in primary care settings compared with teamwork in other organisational settings. Thirdly, we encourage researchers to use research evidence to justify the use of intervention techniques or teambuilding methods. This chapter suggests that the existing enthusiasm for teamwork deserves to be sustained, but needs to be tempered by recognition of the following: effective teamwork is difficult to achieve; the context of primary care (with its hierarchical structures and organisational overlaps) creates particular and difficult challenges; bringing about effective change is not simply a matter of building cohesive teams, but also involves robustly challenging rigid patterns of team and organisational functioning.

Editors' summary

In this chapter, West and Poulton have explored the notion of the team or work group, and have outlined some of the relevant literature. In particular, they have discussed what types of groupings may be thought of as teams, the reasons why people organise work in groups, and some of the problems people encounter when functioning within a group (e.g. in generating ideas or making effective decisions). Drawing on their own recent work, they have then compared primary health care teams with other multidisciplinary teams with regard to four key dimensions of team functioning. They conclude that primary health care team functioning is significantly different to the others tested, with primary health care teams scoring lowest of all the groups on all but one scale. Important suggestions for change are made by West and Poulton. The structural difficulties which they see as a major impediment to the development of effective teamwork are potentially addressed in the 1996 White Paper, *Choice and Opportunity* (Secretary of State for Health, 1996). Further development must take these issues into account.

References

Anderson NR and West MA (1994) *The Team Climate Inventory: Manual and Scoring Guide.* NFER/Nelson, Windsor.

Brown RJ (1988) *Group Processes: Dynamics Within and Between Groups.* Basil Blackwell, London.

Cyert RM and March JE (1963) *A Behavioral Theory of the Firm.* Prentice Hall, Englewood Cliffs.

Darley JM and Latané B (1968) Bystander intervention in emergencies: diffusion of responsibility. *Journal of Personality and Social Psychology* 8, 377–83.

Diehl M and Stroebe W (1987) Productivity loss in brainstorming groups: towards the solution of a riddle. *Journal of Personality and Social Psychology* 53, 497–509.

Field R and West MA (1995) Teamwork in primary health care: perspectives from practices. *Journal of Interprofessional Care* 9, 123–30.

Goodman PS, Raulia EC and Argote L (1986) Correct thinking about groups setting the stage for new ideas. In Goodman PS *et al.* (eds) *Designing Effective Work Groups.* Jossey Bass, San Francisco.

Guzzo RA and Shea GP (1992) Group performance and inter-group relations in organisations. In Dunnette MD and Hough LM (eds) *Handbook of Industrial and Organizational Psychology, Vol. 3,* pp. 269–313. Consulting Psychologists Press, Palo Alto.

Hackman JR (ed.) (1990) *Groups That Work (and Those That Don't). Creating Conditions for Effective Teamwork.* Jossey Bass, San Francisco.

Janis IL (1982) *Groupthink: A Study of Foreign Policy Decisions and Fiascos,* 2nd edn. Houghton Mifflin, Boston.

Latané B, Williams K and Harkins S (1979) Many hands make light work: the causes and consequences of social loafing. *Journal of Personality and Social Psychology* 37, 822–32.

McCauley C (1989) The nature of social influence in groupthink: compliance and internalization. *Journal of Personality and Social Psychology* 57, 250–60.

Myers DG and Lamm H (1976) The group polarization phenomenon. *Psychological Bulletin* 83, 602–27.

Ringelmann M (1913) Recherches sur les moteurs animés: travail de l'homme. *Annales de l'Institut National Agronomique, 2nd Series,* 12, 1–40.

Rogelberg SG, Barnes-Farrell JL and Lower CA (1992) The stepladder technique: an alternative group structure facilitating effective group decision-making. *Journal of Applied Psychology* 77, 730–7.

Secretary of State for Health (1996) *Choice and Opportunity.* The Stationery Office, London (Cm 3390).

Steiner ID (1972) *Group Process and Productivity.* Academic Press, Orlando.

Wall TD and Lischeron JH (1977) *Worker Participation: A Critique of the Evidence and Some Fresh Evidence.* McGraw-Hill, Maidenhead.

Weldon E and Weingart LR (1993) Group goals and group performance. *British Journal of Social Psychology* 32, 307–34.

West MA (1994) *Effective Teamwork.* British Psychological Society, Leicester.

West MA (1996) Reflexivity and work group effectiveness: a conceptual integration. In West MA (ed.) *The Handbook of Work Group Psychology,* pp. 555–76. Wiley, Chichester.

West MA and Poulton BC (1997) Primary health care teams: a failure of function. *Journal of Interprofessional Care,* in press.

3

The changing composition of primary health care teams

Tim Usherwood, Sarah Long and Helen Joesbury

Introduction

Following the introduction of the NHS in 1948, the vast majority of general practitioners in the UK continued to work either single-handed or in small partnerships, with little or no assistance from members of other occupational groups. These days, most general practice teams include several doctors and a wide range of clerical, administrative and other workers. Some of the non-medical workers are employed by the practice, and others are attached to it. What are the changes that have occurred, and why have these changes taken place? The aims of this chapter are to review developments in the composition of practice teams with particular attention to the last few years, to discuss some of the reasons for these changes, and to present some of the implications for health service managers, policy-makers and team members themselves.

Practice teams 1946–1990

Three surveys of general practice in the UK were published during the first decade of the NHS (Collings, 1950; Hadfield, 1953; Taylor, 1954). The majority of practices described in these reports were based on one or two doctors, and about half appear to have employed a full-time or part-time secretary or secretary-receptionist. A smaller proportion employed a practice nurse. In the majority of cases the doctor was male and married, and his wife helped with the practice in a variety of ways. Although the reports mention district nurses, midwives and health visitors, interaction between these workers and the general practitioners is barely discussed. Perhaps significantly, it was not until 1974 that district nurses and health visitors ceased to be employed by local authorities, and were instead employed within the health service.

The report by Collings (1950) was highly critical of UK general practice. The others, too, had recommendations to make. Among these were suggestions for increasing the support available to general practitioners in their practices. However, little or nothing changed until the mid-1960s, when the British Medical Association published its Charter for the Family Doctor Service (British Medical Association, 1965) and, armed with the threat of mass resignations, negotiated a new contract for general practitioners. Relevant aspects of this were payment of a group practice allowance to principals working in a practice with three or more partners, and 70 per cent reimbursement of the salaries of up to two full-time ancillary staff or their part-time equivalents, per principal.

By 1977, Cartwright and Anderson (1981) found that virtually all practices were employing at least one secretary or receptionist, and 84 per cent of the doctors in their sample had at least one nurse working in the practice. The nurses might be employed or attached, or both. The majority of doctors reported attached health visitors, midwives and district nurses, and 23 per cent reported an attached social worker.

At about the same time, Bowling (1981) published a book in which she argued for greater delegation of clinical tasks to nurses by general practitioners. However, she also found, from interviews with doctors and practice nurses, that significant numbers of both groups held unfavourable attitudes to such delegation.

The notion of the primary health care team was sufficiently well established by the early 1980s for the words to appear in the title of a government report (Department of Health and Social Security, 1981). The literature of the time suggests that such teams were seen as including health visitors, midwives, district nurses and other attached workers, as well as the doctors and employees of the practice (Bowling, 1981). However, in 1986 the Cumberlege Report (Department of Health and Social Security, 1986) recommended a change from practice-attached district nurses and health visitors to community nursing teams managed on a neighbourhood basis. This had the potential to weaken the links between practices and community nurses responsible for the care of the same patients. Although many health authorities initially implemented the recommendations, practice-attached nursing teams were subsequently reinstituted.

The situation by 1990, before the introduction of the 'New Contract' for general practice (Department of Health and the Welsh Office, 1989), was that the majority of general practitioners worked in group practices, with employed administrative staff and possibly nurses or other clinical workers, and with attached community nurses, midwives and health visitors. In the next section of this chapter we shall present the findings of research to quantify the composition of practice teams immediately before the 1990 contract was introduced, 1 year later, and 3 years after that.

Practice teams during the period 1990–1994

In 1989, David Hannay proposed a study to investigate changes in the composition of practice teams associated with the introduction of the New Contract in April 1990. This entailed a survey of all practices in Sheffield between February and March 1990, before the introduction of the 1990 contract, and again during the same months in 1991 (Hannay *et al.*, 1992). Between October and November 1994, we repeated this survey as part of a national survey of practice teams (Usherwood *et al.*, 1995).

The sampling frame for the three surveys was the Sheffield Family Health Services Authority (Sheffield FHSA) list of general medical practices. In 1990, and again in 1991, a letter explaining the study was sent to all general practitioners in Sheffield. This was followed with a questionnaire which was sent to each practice. Non-responding practices were sent a single reminder letter. Of the 120 practices in Sheffield during those years, 68 practices (57 per cent) responded in 1990 and 73 practices (61 per cent) responded in 1991.

In 1994, we sent a questionnaire and covering letter to the practice manager or senior receptionist of each practice. We did not send an initial letter to the general practitioners. We sent two reminders to non-responders, and then contacted the practice by telephone. Of the 122 practices on the list that year, 117 practices (96 per cent) responded. The questionnaires for 1990 and 1991 were identical, and the questionnaire for 1994 was modified somewhat but sought the same information.

The mean numbers of different occupational groups reported per practice team in each of the three surveys are listed in Table 3.1. Also listed for groups of employed workers are the mean numbers of full-time equivalents, based on a notional 35-hour week. The latter information is not given for the non-employed occupational groups; it is not relevant for general practitioner principals, and it was not collected for attached workers in the 1990 and 1991 surveys.

It can be seen from the first row of data in Table 3.1 that the mean number of general practitioner principals increased by 0.8 doctors over a period of 4 years, to 3.23 per practice. At least some of this increase probably reflected a rise in the proportions of fractional-time and job-sharing principals. Nevertheless, it did represent an increase in the number of individuals working in the practices, and thus interacting with one another, with other team members, and with patients.

The average team had a total of 4.07, 4.58 and 5.26 full-time equivalent employed administrative workers in 1990, 1991 and 1994, respectively. Table 3.1 shows that most of this increase was accounted for by a rise in the number of receptionists, fund managers and computer operators. Between 1990 and

Table 3.1 Composition of practice teams in Sheffield in 1990, 1991 and 1994

Occupational group	Mean number (mean full-time equivalents) reported per practice		
	1990	1991	1994
GP principals	2.43	2.58	3.23
Employed workers			
Practice managers	0.81 (0.76)	0.78 (0.75)	0.91 (0.88)
Fund managers	Not relevant	See footnote	0.22 (0.16)
Receptionists	3.95 (2.53)	4.32 (2.96)	4.81 (3.35)
Secretaries/typists	0.94 (0.68)	0.83 (0.63)	0.80 (0.56)
Computer operators	0.10 (0.10)	0.29 (0.24)	0.38 (0.31)
Practice nurses	1.70 (1.11)	1.83 (1.13)	1.74 (1.21)
Nurse practitioners	0.03 (0.02)	0.10 (0.07)	0.08 (0.05)
Counsellors/psychologists	0.22 (0.07)	0.23 (0.07)	0.28 (0.08)
Chiropodists	0.00 (0.00)	0.10 (0.01)	0.15 (0.02)
Cleaners	See footnote	See footnote	1.14 (0.34)
Others	0.42 (0.13)	0.46 (0.21)	0.65 (0.31)
Attached workers			
District nurses	2.29	2.18	2.13
Health visitors	1.60	2.11	1.31
Midwives	1.10	1.02	0.97
Social workers	0.57	0.38	0.05
Community psychiatric nurses	1.10	1.05	0.34
Counsellors/psychologists	0.16	0.11	0.02
Physiotherapists	0.52	0.48	See footnote
Chiropodists	0.17	0.21	0.23
Others	0.22	0.15	1.30

Information about certain occupational groups was not collected in all surveys. Team members in these groups were classified within the category 'Others'.

1994, Sheffield FHSA had a policy of investing in practices to increase the numbers of receptionists (G. Rotherham, Sheffield FHSA, personal communication, 1995). Most of the practices that became fundholding after the scheme was introduced in April 1991 appointed fund managers. Only two practices in Sheffield joined the scheme in the first year, but of the 117 respondents in 1994, 31 respondents (26 per cent) were fundholders and a further 11 respondents (9 per cent) were preparing for this step. A substantial management allowance was available to fundholding practices and those preparing for fundholding to enable them to employ additional administrative workers such as fund managers. The cost of employing a computer operator could also be set against this allowance if his or her work is directly related to managing the fund.

Among the employed clinical workers, the main change was a 9 per cent increase between 1990 and 1994 in the mean number of full-time equivalent practice nurses per practice. A national survey of general practitioners undertaken in 1990 showed that 51 per cent of them had already created a new nursing post within their practice in anticipation of the requirements of that year's new contract, and 83 per cent had expanded the role of nurses already employed by them (Robinson *et al.*, 1993). The increase in the number of practice nurses continued after the 1990 contract, both in Sheffield and nationally (Department of Health, 1994).

An average of 7.73, 7.69 and 6.35 workers were attached to the practices in 1990, 1991 and 1994, respectively. The changes were largely due to significant reductions in the number of attached social workers and community psychiatric nurses, and also in the reported number of district nurses, health visitors and midwives. The Sheffield social work department underwent restructuring during this period, with a considerable reduction in attachments to practices. The decreases in the reported number of other attached workers are more difficult to explain. They may have represented reductions in investment, but may also have reflected changes in human resource management policy by the local health service providers who employed these groups of workers (J. Collins, Community Health Sheffield, personal communication, 1995).

England and Wales in 1994

The 1994 Sheffield survey was part of a larger survey that we conducted across the whole of the UK. The sampling processes in Scotland and Northern Ireland were biased in order to over-represent selected geographical areas. However, in England and Wales we selected a representative sample via a two-stage process. A total of 24 Family Health Services Authorities (FHSAs) were selected at random from a total of 98 FHSAs in the two countries. We contacted each FHSA that was selected and asked them for a list of general practices which they administered. All of the FHSAs responded. We then drew a 20 per cent random sample from the list of each FHSA, and in this way identified a total of 505 practices across England and Wales.

The survey process was exactly the same as that described above for Sheffield practices, except that we did not telephone all non-respondents. Instead, we selected non-respondents for telephoning at random until we achieved a response rate of over 80 per cent. We also offered those practice managers/receptionists whom we telephoned the opportunity to respond to the questionnaire over the telephone. In the end, 409 (81 per cent) practices responded. Of these, 386 responses were returned by mail and 23 responses were obtained by telephone.

The median list size of the responding practices was in the range 5000–9999. Ninety-six responding practices (23 per cent) were fundholding, and 38 practices (9 per cent) were preparing to fundhold in 1995. A total of

119 respondents (29 per cent) were training practices, and 70 respondents (17 per cent) were dispensing. A total of 359 practices (88 per cent), including all of the fundholders, had a computerized repeat-prescribing system.

The mean numbers of different occupational groups reported per practice team are listed in the first column of Table 3.2, and the mean number of full-time equivalents (FTE) are given in brackets, based on a notional 35-hour week. Responding practices had a mean number of 3.22 general practitioner principals, 11.80 employed workers (7.37 FTE) and 6.33 attached workers (3.19 FTE).

The second column of Table 3.2 shows the median numbers of each occupational group that were reported per practice, and the final column shows the range of numbers of each group per practice. It can be seen from the last column that, apart from general practitioner principals, no single occupational group was represented in all of the responding practices. On the other hand, a wide range of different groups was reported by the

Table 3.2 Composition of practice teams in England and Wales in 1994

Occupational group	Number reported per practice		
	Mean (FTE)	Median	Range
GP principals	3.22	3	1–11
Employed workers			
Practice managers	0.93 (0.89)	1	0–2
Fund managers	0.16 (0.13)	0	0–2
Receptionists	5.08 (3.37)	5	0–18
Secretaries/typists	1.01 (0.65)	1	0–7
Computer operators	0.44 (0.32)	0	0–6
Practice nurses	1.94 (1.21)	2	0–7
Nurse practitioners	0.04 (0.03)	0	0–2
Counsellors/psychologists	0.20 (0.03)	0	0–3
Chiropodists	0.02 (0.00)	0	0–2
Cleaners	0.99 (0.26)	1	0–6
Others	1.02 (0.38)	—	—
Attached workers			
District nurses	1.82 (1.37)	2	0–9
Nurse auxiliaries	0.54 (0.24)	0	0–4
Health visitors	1.44 (1.02)	1	0–5
Midwives	0.96 (0.33)	1	0–8
Social workers	0.09 (0.01)	0	0–6
Community psychiatric nurses	0.45 (0.10)	0	0–6
Counsellors/psychologists	0.09 (0.01)	0	0–3
Chiropodists	0.21 (0.02)	0	0–4
Others	0.76 (0.15)	—	—

FTE, full-time equivalent.

practices. A total of 41 groups of employed workers were listed on the questionnaire or included by respondents in the category 'Other', while 36 different groups of attached workers were identified in the same way.

When interpreting these data, we found it helpful to adopt the notion of a 'typical practice team', which we defined as consisting of the median numbers of those occupational groups which were represented in the majority of responding teams. From the second column of Table 3.2, therefore, a typical responding practice team consisted of three general practitioner principals, one practice manager, five receptionists (one of whom was a senior receptionist), one secretary/typist, two practice nurses, one cleaner, two district nurses, one health visitor and one midwife.

The notion of a typical practice team is elaborated further in Table 3.3. The first column of data is a tabulation of the typical team of all respondents. The second and third columns show the typical teams of large and small responding practices, respectively. Large practices were those that reported 5000 or more patients, and small practices reported less than 5000 patients. A typical large practice team included members of the same occupational groups as that based on all practices, but had more doctors, receptionists and health visitors. A typical small practice team had fewer doctors, receptionists, practice nurses and district nurses, and also lacked a secretary.

The last two columns of Table 3.3 allow comparison of fundholding and non-fundholding practices. Fundholding practices were larger on average than non-fundholders, and a typical fundholding team had more doctors, receptionists, practice nurses, district nurses and health visitors. In addition, a typical fundholding team included a fund manager, while exactly 50 per cent of the responding fundholding practices reported that they had a computer operator.

Discussion

At the inception of the NHS the typical practice team consisted of one or two doctors and perhaps an employed administrative worker. Some practices also employed a nurse, although most did not. District nurses and health visitors were employed by the local authority and did not appear to interact significantly with local general practitioners, except perhaps occasionally in relation to individual patients. We have found little information about interaction with midwives, although those doctors who undertook domiciliary midwifery must have formed working relationships with members of this occupational group, then as now.

By 1994, the typical practice team was up to three doctors in strength and had expanded almost beyond all recognition in terms of employed administrative staff and employed and attached clinical workers. What have been the reasons for these developments, and what are the implications?

Table 3.3 Composition of typical practice teams

Occupational group	Median number reported per practice				
	All practices	Large practices	Small practices	Fundholding	Non-fundholding
GP principals	3	4	2	4	2
Employed workers					
Practice managers	1	1	1	1	1
Fund managers	0	0	0	1	0
Senior receptionist	1	1	1	1	1
Other receptionists	4	6	2	5	3
Secretary/typist	1	1	0	1	1
Computer operators	0	0	0	0.5	0
Practice nurses	2	2	1	3	2
Cleaners	1	1	1	1	1
Attached workers					
District nurses	2	2	1	2	1
Health visitors	1	2	1	2	1
Midwives	1	1	1	1	1

Only occupational groups represented in one or more typical practice teams are listed here.

Where there is a difference in the table between large and small practices, or between fundholders and non-fundholders, this reached the level of statistical significance (median test; $P < 0.001$ in all cases).

Four groups of factors appear to have been significant in influencing changes in the composition of practice teams:

- health service investment policies;
- legal and contractual requirements;
- cultural changes;
- technological developments.

Health service investment policies

The ability and willingness of FHSAs (and Family Practitioner Committees before 1990) to invest in practice teams has been a major influence on the latter's growth over the last 30 years. The introduction in 1966 of 70 per cent reimbursement of the salaries of up to two full-time equivalent ancillary staff per principal was followed by a substantial increase in the numbers of employed workers. A group practice allowance was introduced at the same time, payable to principals working in a partnership of three or more, and this was followed by an increase in the proportion of such partnerships. More recently, a management allowance became available to fundholding practices in order to meet the costs of employing staff to assist in the administration of the fund; most fundholding practices have employed a fund manager, and in 1994 approximately 50 per cent employed a computer operator.

It is not just the numbers of partners and employed workers that have been affected by health service investment policies. Investment decisions have also influenced the numbers of workers attached to practices. The decision during the 1970s by Health Authorities to employ nurses and to place them in practices enhanced the composition of practice teams at that time (Cartwright and Anderson, 1981). Since the construction of an internal market within the health service, decisions by purchasers have led providers to review their investment in numbers, grades and working hours of district nurses, midwives, health visitors and community psychiatric nurses (J. Collins, Community Health Sheffield, personal communication, 1995).

Legal and contractual requirements

Of course, the availability of funds is not the only factor that influences investment in human resources in the general practice (Bosanquet and Leese, 1986). Changes in the legal and contractual context may also have had an effect on the composition of teams. In their 1990 survey, cited above, Robinson *et al.* (1993) found that 50 per cent of the responding general practitioners had created a new nursing post within their practice in anticipation of the requirements of the 1990 contract, and over 75 per cent had expanded the role of the nurses already employed. As an example, one of the new requirements was that general practitioners offered all registered patients aged 75 years and over a consultation for health promotional purposes. In a survey of practice undertaken during the year following the introduction of the contract, Ross *et al.* (1994) found that over 68 per cent of nurses undertook these health checks on behalf of their practices.

Cultural changes

A third factor in the development of practice teams seems likely to have been changes in the culture of general practice, the health service, and the society of which they are a part. Thus the expectations of general practitioners with regard to their lifestyle may have contributed to the increasing proportion of group practices over the last 30 years; it is easier to arrange holidays and so forth in a partnership. Another example is provided by the growing number of counsellors in general practice. This growth may reflect changes in patients' expectations of services that should be available to them, and changes in doctors' views of what services should be provided.

Technological developments

Finally, there have been enormous developments in technology since the NHS was founded. In Sheffield in 1990, only 46 per cent of responding practices had a computer. By 1994, 95 per cent had a computerized repeat-prescribing system. Concurrently, the proportion of practices which reported having an employed computer operator increased from under 10 per cent in 1990 to 28 per cent in 1994.

The four groups of factors identified above have not, of course, operated independently of one another. For example, most vaccines against infectious diseases have been developed in the last 50 years – a technological development. This has led to the expectation within society that children will be offered appropriate protection – a cultural change. Protocols for childhood immunisation have been developed, and a practice undertaking such immunisations is subject to legal and contractual requirements. All three factors are likely to influence decisions concerning financial investment in practice teams, and thus to affect their composition.

Implications for the future

What are the implications of the issues raised in this chapter for the future of practice team development? Clearly, governments have the opportunity to influence the composition of teams through a combination of legal and fiscal policy. However, these are relatively blunt and unwieldy instruments; an increase in recruitment of practice nurses by general practitioners in anticipation of the 1990 contract was not necessarily foreseen or foreseeable.

Similarly, FHSAs have the opportunity to influence the numbers and types of workers employed by practices through selective investment policies. Purchasers, both commissioning authorities and fundholding practices, can influence the numbers and types of attached workers through the contracts that they negotiate with the relevant providers.

At a practice level, the fact that a team includes workers from a wide variety of employed and attached occupational groups provides a great challenge in terms of management and leadership. On the one hand, the team contains workers with a range of potentially conflicting professional allegiances, values and contractual responsibilities. On the other hand, these workers are responsible for the care of substantially overlapping groups of patients, and for working together in providing that care. The task of the practice team is to provide effective care that is relevant to the needs of the community it serves, is accessible to all members of that community, and is delivered as efficiently as possible in order to maximise the benefits obtained from the available human and other resources. We do not yet know the optimal composition for a practice team serving any particular community, but we do know that if team members are to achieve these goals, then they must share a common vision and underpinning values (West, 1994), they must critically reflect on their own practice (Schon, 1987), and they must engage in constant, open dialogue with one another and with the members of the community that they serve (Bryant, 1988; Brown, 1994).

Such processes depend upon two factors. The practice needs to provide structured opportunities for personal, professional and organisational development (Usherwood, 1993). In addition, these opportunities must both inform and be informed by a culture in which questioning and debate are facilitated, valued and taken seriously by every member of the team (Argyris and Schon, 1978; Senge, 1990).

Editors' summary

This chapter has demonstrated how useful longitudinal research can be in describing change. Usherwood and his colleagues have described the evolution of primary health care teams in the UK, drawing on an initial study based in one district prior to the introduction of the 1990 Contract for General Practice (Department of Health and the Welsh Office, 1989), and a follow-up study which compared the later situation in that district with a wider sample drawn from across the UK. They have identified four groups of factors which they believe have influenced the changes described, namely investment policies, contractual requirements, cultural changes and technological development. They indicate that the operation of these factors has not been predictable to date. It is not clear what the optimum team membership or size might be. However, the authors conclude by stressing the importance of promoting a culture of team and individual development in order to optimise effectiveness.

References

Argyris C and Schon D (1978) *Organisational Learning*. Addison Wesley, Reading, MA.

Bosanquet N and Leese B (1986) Family doctors; their choice of practice strategy. *British Medical Journal* 293, 667–70.

Bowling A (1981) *Delegation in General Practice*. Tavistock, London.

British Medical Association (1965) A charter for the family doctor service. *British Medical Journal Supplement* 1, 89–91.

Brown I (1994) Community and participation for general practice: perceptions of general practitioners and community nurses. *Social Science and Medicine* 39, 335–44.

Bryant J (1988) Reflections at the midpoint on progress and prospects. In *From Alma-Ata to the Year 2000*. World Health Organization, Geneva.

Cartwright A and Anderson R (1981) *General Practice Revisited*. Tavistock, London.

Collings JS (1950) General practice in England today. *Lancet* 1, 555–85.

Department of Health (1994) *Statistics for General Medical Practitioners in England and Wales: 1983–1993*. Department of Health, Leeds.

Department of Health and Social Security (1981) *The Primary Health Care Team. Report by a Joint Working Group of the Standing Medical Advisory Committee and the Standing Nursing and Midwifery Advisory Committee*. HMSO, London.

Department of Health and Social Security (1986) *Neighbourhood Nursing – a Focus for Care. Report of the Community Nursing Review*. HMSO, London.

Department of Health and the Welsh Office (1989) *General Practice in the National Health Service. A New Contract*. HMSO, London.

Hadfield SJ (1953) A field survey of general practice 1951–1952. *British Medical Journal* 2, 683–706.

Hannay DR, Usherwood TP and Platts M (1992) Practice organisation before and after a new contract: a survey of general practice in Sheffield. *British Journal of General Practice* 42, 517–20.

Robinson G, Beaton S and White P (1993) Attitudes towards practice nurses – survey of a sample of general practitioners in England and Wales. *British Journal of General Practice* 43, 25–9.

Ross FM, Bower PJ and Sibbald BS (1994) Practice nurses: characteristics, workload and training needs. *British Journal of General Practice* 44, 15–18.

Schon D (1987) *Educating the Reflective Practitioner*. Jossey-Bass, San Francisco.

Senge P (1990) *The Fifth Discipline*. Doubleday, New York.

Taylor S (1954) *Good General Practice*, Oxford University Press, London.

Usherwood T (1993) The primary care organisation: team or hologram? *Journal of Interprofessional Care* 7, 211–16.

Usherwood T, Barker S and Joesbury H (1995) *Primary Health Care Teams in Britain*. Unpublished report to the Department of Employment, Sheffield, and the NHS Executive, Leeds.

West M (1994) *Effective Teamwork*. British Psychological Society, Leicester.

Acknowledgements

We wish to thank Professor David Hannay for permission to report findings from the 1990 and 1991 Sheffield survey database, and the Employment Department and NHS Executive for their support of the 1994 national survey. The views expressed in this chapter are those of the authors.

4

Working in the wider team

Sheila Edward

Introduction

This chapter will look at personal informal solutions, adopted by individual professionals, to the problem of multiprofessional teamwork in the community, as opposed to formal solutions worked out through planned collaboration among team members or implemented as part of a management or training strategy.

It is based on a 3-year qualitative investigation into the personal concepts of staff membership, development and practice of a range of professionals working in multiprofessional settings in North-East England, including nurses, doctors, social workers, teachers, physiotherapists, occupational therapists, dietitians, speech therapists, chiropodists and nursery nurses. Loosely structured interviews were conducted with 103 staff in the following four settings:

- a special school where many children needed continuing care and therapy, both from school-based nursing and physiotherapy teams and from visiting professionals;
- a community nursery in a deprived area, selected to allow investigation of collaboration between nursery staff and local community professionals, especially health visitors and social workers;
- the general medical directorate of a district hospital, focusing on collaboration between rehabilitation staff and ward teams of nurses and doctors;
- the elderly care directorate of that hospital, chosen on the assumption that the longer average hospital stay of elderly patients and the more complex problems which they present might have implications for multiprofessional teamworking.

The interviews were supplemented by observation at multiprofessional meetings. Of particular interest were the ways in which professionals shared information when there were no formal structures or rules for teamworking, and their perceptions of the roles of other professionals who were involved with their clients. This chapter draws primarily on data collected in the first two settings, although the interviews with hospital staff helped to put the community data into perspective.

A different perspective on teamwork

Because this research is concerned with a wider range of professionals – including, but not limited to, members of primary health care teams – and focuses on individual experience rather than on managerial definitions of team effectiveness, this chapter does not share all of the underlying assumptions of the preceding and following chapters. For example, West and Poulton in Chapter 2, and again, Freake and van Zwanenberg in Chapter 7, define teams in terms which do not fit the broader interpretation of team-working in the community which will be discussed here. These two types of teamworking differ in two important aspects.

First, shared objectives cannot be taken for granted in the contexts discussed here. All members of the group of professionals providing services to a common client may not share objectives with regard to their work, beyond the broad intention of contributing to the well-being of the client – an objective which is so general that it leaves plenty of room for debate over the nature of the professional interventions which will lead to its achievement. Some professionals may view the clients' medical needs as paramount, while others consider that their emotional or educational needs have priority, and where several professions are involved in the education and care of, for example, a child with physical disabilities, there is potential for disharmony. Where the objectives of the group's work are disputed, 'social loafing' (West and Poulton, 1997) becomes less of a problem than conflict resolution (Nason, 1983) or rival claims to client advocacy (Webb, 1987). Perhaps we can only speculate about the outcome if Ringelmann's (1913) rope-pulling experiment (see Chapter 2) was to be repeated, this time not with seven team members pulling in one direction, but with three pulling in one direction and four in another, although it seems likely that the outcome would satisfy no one. The problem of agreeing upon team objectives is further complicated by the commitment of many social services, education and health professionals to helping clients to define and achieve their own goals, which may be at odds with the goals that other professionals have defined for them. Thus the research interest in this context was to discover how aware interviewees were of the objectives of other professionals working with clients, and whether they attempted to influence one another, to align objectives or to accommodate differing beliefs about clients' needs.

Secondly, professionals did not necessarily see themselves as members of a formal team, although the roles and interactions which they described fitted well with Øvretveit's definition of a community multidisciplinary team as 'a small group of people, usually from different professions and agencies, who relate to each other to contribute to the common goal of meeting the health and social needs of one client, or those of a client population in the community' (Øvretveit, 1993). The key clause in this definition is *'who relate to each other'*. Øvretveit, in common with many participants in this project, stresses the importance of the relationships between professionals, and between professional and client: 'These relationships are not secondary to the goal of the team, as they are in some project teams in industry, but are the means through which the client is helped' (Øvretveit, 1993).

The conditions in a complex community team are not always propitious for the building of interprofessional relationships. The full range of professionals contributing to the provision of services to a common client may never all meet together. They may not see themselves as a defined or bounded group in the way that a functional group within an organisation may be described. Moreover, the size of the group is often larger than the 'maximum effective team size' of 8 to 12 members, simply because clients' needs are complex and require input from a large and fluctuating number of different agencies and professionals. Whereas staffing of practice teams, as described in Chapter 3, is relatively stable and drawn from a limited range of professions and occupations, the shape and composition of the wider team and the personnel involved in case conferences or care teams change constantly. Such change might occur in response to the needs of the particular client around whom the team is centred. For example, a child protection case might draw in teachers and other professionals involved with older siblings of a nursery-age child at risk. The shape of the team may also be altered by changes in legislation or redefinition of professional responsibilities, as in *Working Together Under the Children Act 1989* (Home Office Department of Health, Department of Education and Science and the Welsh Office, 1991), or by changes in the structure or premises of any uniprofessional team, such as reorganisation of patch-based social workers into a unified team covering a broad area, obliging each social worker to develop wider, more geographically dispersed networks in place of the local, more frequent contacts of the patch system. Nevertheless, despite the communication difficulties inherent in network teams with their fluctuating memberships, channels of communication *do* open and relationships *are* built. Key questions in this research concerned the extent to which the individual professionals were aware of, and valued, the contributions of others, and how they collaborated informally or formally to co-ordinate their practice.

Because this was a qualitative ethnographic project, the researcher's personal viewpoint must be clarified. Although supported by a research team of experienced practitioners in education, nursing and social work, the author is an outsider to each of the professions discussed here, rather than an insider practitioner-researcher (Reed and Procter, 1995). This perspective may be an advantage when researching interprofessional issues, since the interviewer clearly cannot be an insider to each of many professions. My own relevant academic knowledge base is in personnel management, but this was acquired relatively recently, following a career change after 16 years of working in complex organisations, without benefit of formal theories of management, organisational behaviour or employee development. I therefore draw not only on the 'propositional knowledge' (Eraut, 1994) of those disciplines, but also on personal knowledge and interpretation of previous experience in a variety of employment roles – as autonomous professional, as manager and, most relevantly, as a member or leader of many workplace teams with varying degrees of cohesion, awareness, task orientation and effectiveness. In short, I came to this project with Belbin (1993) and other theorists of team and organisational behaviour in my toolkit, but also with a partly experientially based suspicion that even in situations where managerially led teambuilding initiatives were not in place, individual staff might be adapting their practice and negotiating their roles to fit in with colleagues and to meet their clients' needs.

This is certainly not to disparage formal training policies and events – which may indeed be the ideal approach to improving teamworking in many contexts – but simply to acknowledge that in complex inter-agency networks, where teams may be large and individuals are members of many different client-centred teams, formal teambuilding events may not always be practicable. Nor would I deny the value of job descriptions and clearly defined roles for team members, although Strauss *et al.* (1963) and subsequent writers on 'negotiated order' confirm that the paperwork defining roles does not always reflect everyday practice. A better understanding of individuals' practical, personal strategies for working together, and of the conditions which are favourable to such strategies, may suggest ways in which managers can encourage good practice in future.

Cross-professional values and shared concerns in the community

It would have been possible to analyse the data by profession, looking for differences between the values and approaches to teamworking of, say, health visitors and social workers. Instead, the following analysis seeks first to illustrate common ground in professionals' approaches to their work, before exploring in the discussion how these values influence the processes of formal multiprofessional working. Three important themes emerged across the spectrum of professionals interviewed in community settings, namely flexibility, accessibility (both to clients and to one another), and valuing the contributions of other professionals.

Flexibility

Much evidence was obtained of willingness to interpret professional roles flexibly, and to accept a complex, rather than narrow, interpretation of responsibilities. This flexibility was frequently described as stemming from client needs. For example, within the school environment, children had the services of nurses and physiotherapists, but the whole team could not accompany the teachers on educational excursions:

> Say, for example, teachers weren't prepared to administer medication or dress children or put calipers on or off, they wouldn't go anywhere. .... I think it is like your own family, you do things for your own children if you are with them, and I think if you are away with children, you take on that role of the parents and do what needs to be done for them.
>
> (Teacher in special school)

Physiotherapists, too, acknowledged a role that included social and emotional support to children and their families:

> One of our physiotherapy students who came on a third year placement made the comment at the end 'Well, it was a great placement, but there's not a lot of physiotherapy that goes on.' That was interesting because what else can you do? We do a lot of talking, a lot of advising, a lot of liaison and so on. But it has become very specialised: we obviously do do the nitty-gritty, the treatment, hands-on, but there is a lot more to it.
>
> (Physiotherapist in special school)

A health visitor working on a deprived housing estate described adapting her daily work to fit the needs of the patch:

> I think possibly specifically with working here, I spend a lot of time liaising with social workers, which I never did in my previous post; and I spend a lot of time on the telephone to Housing and loan equipment places and organising bags of clothes, rather than going in to people and saying, 'Let's do this developmental check-up . . .'
>
> (Health visitor)

Counselling, even just giving time to listen, became part of the role of many professionals:

> Some of the things that they talk about have got nothing to do with housing management proper – it's more to do with what is happening on the estate and the fears and problems that they have.
>
> (Community housing manager)

Accepting a broader role could, however, sometimes conflict with meeting the narrower requirements of the prime professional role:

> Not only do you have the physical disabilities, but we've got the emotional problems as well, which we try to take into account when we have a class in front of us. But very often, if you have an emotional outburst, then that is the

lesson finished: you spend a lot of your time dealing with that one child. It's difficult really.

(Teacher in special school)

Even a health visitor, who described her role primarily in terms of liaison with other professionals, and who regularly put clients in touch with colleagues or specialists who might be able to help with a specific problem, found the sheer breadth of her role, or at least client expectations of her role, stressful at times:

> I find a lot of my visits are for children who are doing all right and I see them and everything is hunky-dory, but then maybe the next 40 minutes are taken up with some sort of social issues, say the partners have split up and they are worried about money and they need help with getting re-housed or whatever, and that bothers me a bit because I don't feel very equipped to deal with that, and sometimes I find that very frustrating.

(Health visitor)

This echoes the findings of Rowe *et al.* (1995) with regard to the impact of vulnerable families on the workload of health visitors. Several different professions noted recent changes in the balance of work in the community. Social workers regretted the loss of flexibility in their casework following the Children Act 1989 (Department of Health, 1989), and the increased proportion of statutory work on their caseloads:

> The informal preventative social work no longer exists. In many ways it's the caseloads we are carrying, in terms of, it is all child protection, court work. You feel more like you are policing people now. It feels that you are chasing your tail, you are in and out of court all the time, you are not having the time to do the kind of social work that you want to do – the getting in there, spending time with people, the advising.

(Social worker)

Other professionals, including health visitors and nursery nurses, confirmed that some non-statutory work which they were currently handling might, in more leisurely times, have been covered by social workers. In most cases this was accepted as inevitable, although regrettable:

> We are in a preventative role and although a lot of them in the past would have been referred to social services in prevention, now you have almost got to have definite problems that you can identify and it has got to be enough to be a referral, things have really got to be so bad that they will pick it up. I mean, we do make referrals to Social Services, at least it has been done, it's down on paper and it has been done, but they may not pick it up. I mean things like perhaps childminding – not so much housing problems, but where housing problems are affecting the children, that sort of thing, although perhaps in the past they may have been able to do more . . .

(Health visitor)

Nursery nurses, in particular those specialising in work with families on parenting skills and offering outreach services in the home, were well placed to offer flexible services which social workers and health visitors, with their larger caseloads and their more threatening professional image, might be unable to provide:

> I think that the work I do is non-threatening to parents, and nearly every social worker that I have worked with has said that – that is the valuable part of my contribution, that I can make, I can do an assessment for the social worker in a non-threatening way and build a relationship with the parents. Quite often parents feel very, very threatened by the social worker, so I tend to get a lot more information, although the parent is clear that this information is going to be passed on, but it is confidential, between professionals. ... It is the time factor, you know: social workers have very, very large caseloads and very little time to spend with the people that they are working with, so I have more time to observe the family.
>
> (Nursery nurse/outreach worker)

This 'non-threatening' nursery nurse was providing outreach services to families with either health or social needs – support services which appeared to fit the definition in the *Children Act Report, 1992* of 'acceptable non-stigmatised responses to the normal problems of family life' (Department of Health, 1993, p. 33). Nevertheless, she was also sharing the monitoring role with the other professionals who saw the family less frequently, and with whom she maintained regular, informal contact:

> From an outreach like that, it means that the people who are going to do it, the social worker or the health visitor, I know them and very often it is the same health visitor that you get and so you can build up quite a nice working relationship where you can ring them and say 'I'm not sure about this, I have a gut feeling', because very often you have nothing, it's just a feeling that you get, and I can speak to the health visitor and see. And very often they will ring you as well.
>
> (Nursery nurse/outreach worker)

Social workers spoke appreciatively of the value of others' contributions:

> Where we do use the nursery, health visitors, outreach workers are excellent at taking that pressure away from the social work field role. ... You can't spend the time observing the child and the mother, because of caseload commitments. ... You can't do it alone, there is not any way that you could do this work alone now without the support of others.
>
> (Social worker)

Many other examples could be provided of flexible working in these network teams. Some could be described as boundary-crossing, taking on responsibilities which, strictly speaking, could be seen as the business of another profession, or attempting to influence the practice of a different professional by discussing the needs of a shared client and suggesting ways of meeting those needs collaboratively. In the school, for example, teachers took advice from physiotherapists on the positioning of a child with a physical disability in the classroom, and physiotherapists reinforced the work of the speech therapist. Members of all of the professions, education, health and social work, expressed some responsibility for the emotional needs of the children and said that they discussed their concerns with members of the other professions who were working in the school. In the community team centred around the nursery, the roles of outreach worker, health visitor and social worker appeared to overlap, and almost to merge, around issues of advising and supporting parents. Each professional could describe their own role and the limitations of their own skills with families, yet showed awareness that in fulfilling their role they might obtain information or raise questions about the welfare of the children or families which needed to be shared with other colleagues in the wider team. Boundary disputes – complaints about other team members encroaching on a professional's territory or taking over their role – were conspicuous by their absence.

Accessibility

Three aspects of accessibility were raised in the interviews: accessibility to the public, to clients; accessibility of information; and accessibility of professionals to one another.

In the school setting, the timetable of access to multiprofessional support was managed by the education team. The class teachers were in a position analogous to that of the ward nurses in the hospital, who managed the 24-hour care of the patients, but anticipated that, at negotiated times, other professionals would intervene to assess and treat those patients. In order to avoid excessive disruption to children's education, school-based physio-therapists and nurses arranged their regular sessions as far as possible around the school timetable. Visits from externally based specialists, such as chiropodists or orthotists, were more difficult to timetable, but the principle of negotiating with the teacher before removing the child from class was well established.

This pattern applied only in term-time. Out of term, children who needed regular physiotherapy had access to physiotherapists through home visits. Although all of the professions aimed to build working relationships with the children's parents and to make themselves available to discuss their children's health and educational progress with them, social workers and those who could make home visits appeared to be more accessible to families than the class teachers, partly because teachers lacked space in their working day to develop these relationships. Some teachers said that they valued the opportunity to discuss children in their classes with those who had more insight into the family background. However, opportunities for such discussions were also influenced by the pattern of each professional's working day. Teachers' classroom responsibilities and physiotherapists' part-time contracts prevented their attendance at weekly multiprofessional meetings, where nursing and social work staff met with a representative of the physiotherapist team and the headteacher, representing the education staff, to discuss issues and individual children who were giving cause for concern. Reports of issues discussed at the meeting were fed back to the full teaching and physiotherapist teams at their respective uniprofessional meetings, but interviews revealed that this formal structure for teamwork was widely supplemented by informal 'corridor conferences', brief consultations between class teacher, physiotherapist, nurse and social worker, in which observations or anxieties about the children's behaviour, needs or progress were shared.

In the community team centred around the nursery, accessibility was also valued. The social work team had recently been restructured, moving from a patch-based team system to a children's service team covering half the borough, and withdrawing from a building easily accessible to the local public to a more remote office which housed the majority of the social workers employed in the borough. Although recognising the benefits of working more closely with other colleagues within the profession, a social worker assessed the cost of the change in terms of loss of accessibility:

> I think we have lost a lot. . . . We used to have patch-based health visitors as well as social workers, as well as we shared the building with the police and housing as well. And the schools ... we had developed very, very close working relationships, we knew everybody. That has gone now to a degree, ... instead of working very closely with a few professionals, we are now working less closely with a lot of other professionals and we are spread. ... We are now forming new relationships with different people. You may only have to call in once in a while instead of it being a regular daily contact, so I think in many ways it is a shame we have lost that. Things tend to come in more now at crisis point, whereas before the public could access us, access the other agencies involved much more easily and a quick 10 minutes talk downstairs in one of the rooms could achieve much more.
>
> (Social worker)

Health visitors, meanwhile, remained accessible to the public:

> You need an appointment to see everybody else, but you can always come in off the street and ask to see a health visitor. There is a health visitor with every GP practice and everybody has a right to see one.
>
> (Health visitor)

A social worker acknowledged the knock-on effect of their own withdrawal from the patch:

> And yes, I am sure that health visitors that are still out there and are accessible to the public are having to take on some of the social work role.
>
> (Social worker)

A major cost of changing from a patch-based system was the loss of close daily contact with members of other professions. Other professionals explained the benefits of such contacts, not only for focused work with specific shared clients on their caseload, but also for less focused, more serendipitous information exchange, and for building understanding and relationships that would underpin more formal working together. A recent recruit analysed her approach:

> I am trying very hard to develop, to foster very good working relationships with all the professionals that I need, because, I think, as well as formal information giving, if you build up good networks with individuals, it is very much an informal information giving and receiving system and when you are new to a job, that is something that you are not party to for a long time. I had very good networks where I was before. You used to find out lots of things and not only about individual families, but things that you would work at. You would maybe get to know a council worker and they would say 'Oh yes, they are going to build a park there next year.' Or you would find out that Housing were going to knock down a whole row of houses, which was going to change the community you were working in, and it is information like that. You can prepare yourself for a potential change in practice, you know, if you can get information from elsewhere.
>
> (Health visitor)

Establishing and maintaining contact with members of other professional teams did present challenges. Case conferences on child protection cases might bring together as many as 20 individuals with information on different aspects of the family's life, including social workers, health visitors, nursery nurses or teachers, schoolteachers (if the family included older children), headteachers, school nurses, general practitioners, hospital and community paediatricians, police and, of course, the child's parents. While social workers described going to considerable lengths to stay in touch with all of the relevant parties, particularly in the lead-up to a court case or de-registration conference, others said that they would have appreciated more communication from these more distant network members:

> It is very infrequently that a nursery teacher will ring up. It is usually that we ring them and they have got a vast amount of knowledge of these children because they are seeing them on a daily basis. ... They could perhaps pick things up and let us know what is happening. Usually it is me ringing them up and saying, 'This is what is happening at home: how have they been in the nursery?'
>
> (Health visitor)

Good, regular communication was highly valued, and most of the central members of the care teams interviewed – health visitors, social workers and nursery nurses – felt that their networks worked well. However, a few instances of perceived failure of network members to communicate were noted. The following example highlights the point that it is communication and the relationships between professionals which actually *create* the team:

> I had one case where, in care proceedings, I was getting more information from the foster mother than I was from the social worker; she wasn't even liaising to find out what the health problems were for this little one, she didn't ring me.

That is an extreme case, perhaps, but in that family I did not feel that I was part of a care team. When the social workers do communicate with you, you feel you are part of a care team and you can work together and it also prevents, if you are working together, it prevents the family playing one off against the other, which obviously can happen.

(Health visitor)

Others described past difficulties in developing trusting, information-sharing relationships, problems which had since been overcome:

Initially one health visitor was always thrifty with the information that she would give us, and in fact it might be about children who were on the at-risk register, and I just had to make it clear that staff would not be able to understand and deal with these children, if they didn't have the full picture of their home circumstances, so we have overcome that and I think it is just that they have accepted that we are professionals in our own right, you know, and do a reasonable job.

(Nursery manager)

What are the conditions under which good networking relationships flourish, and professionals learn to see beyond the stereotypes of 'social worker', 'health visitor', 'police officer', 'nursery nurse', etc., and accept them as their colleagues in the team? In this setting, formal multiprofessional training sessions on child protection legislation had played some part, by providing opportunities for staff to meet and to get to know one another:

Putting faces to names is very useful, because they usually try and do it [training] within the locality you are working in, so that the people you are doing the training with, you may come into contact with, and if you have done the course together, it does make it that bit easier.

(Health visitor)

Other factors that were identified as being helpful included sharing premises (which facilitated informal contact and opportunities to get to know other professionals as people), being willing to share information and to listen to and respect other professional viewpoints and, above all, having a chance to work together with shared clients. An excellent opportunity to watch a multiprofessional team in action in a busy nursery arose by chance during the research, and it provided a lively contrast to the formality of case conferences where separate professionals provide their several reports. A central figure in the team subsequently gave her perspective on this integrated work, this opportunity to share experience across professional boundaries and subsequently to discuss their work:

I think this kind of setting is a base for an interdisciplinary assessment, a multidisciplinary assessment. ... This morning has been the ideal situation, you have seen it. The health visitor concerned was there, the speech therapist, the teacher for the visually impaired, the staff who are working with the children in the nursery classroom and the parents – I should put the parents first on the list – we have all been together and that is the beauty of being able to come to a base like this.

(Visiting teacher for the visually impaired)

Perhaps making one's own professional skills and knowledge accessible to colleagues with a different training is one of the greatest challenges for multiprofessional teams. The same teacher made a strong case for openness in professional practice, expressing a preference for working with children in the main classroom, rather than taking them away for assessment in privacy, 'because I think then you are sharing what you are doing with the staff. I'm into demystification, really, not increasing the mystique of it, because we can build on that.' Other instances of openness in professional practice leading to interprofessional learning and practice development included social workers who valued the opportunity to watch nursery nurses working with parents on the development of parenting skills, because they could then reinforce the nursery nurses' work if similar issues arose during social work visits to families at home.

Valuing the contributions of others

Unsurprisingly, members of all professions interviewed said that they valued teamwork and the contributions of their multiprofessional colleagues. The contribution of the nursery staff, for example, was frequently cited with appreciation:

The actual in-depth work you don't have time to do. It's not because we don't want to do it, the time is just not there to do it; which is why the likes of our family centres and our child and family psychiatry are so important to us. It is actually a great sense of relief, certainly from my point of view, knowing you can get a service. ... We often have schools monitoring situations and then contacting us, and health visitors as well.

(Social worker)

Obviously the nursery staff would do their assessment and I am more involved with the child at home. . . . I will go into the nurseries to see them in the nursery setting; but I rely on the nursery staff to do that bit of the assessment, which is in far more detail than I can do, because they have got the families there for the whole day.

(Health visitor)

In general, nursery staff who had undertaken outreach work or given evidence in court in child protection cases did feel that their contribution was valued in the multiprofessional team, and that they were listened to respectfully in case conferences and care-team meetings. They acknowledged receipt of support, encouragement and even praise for their court reports and evidence, from colleagues and senior members of other professions as well as their own. However, other nursery nurses who were based primarily in the day-care nursery had rather less contact with, and feedback from, external professionals. The following quotation from a nursery-based officer suggests that there is only a fine dividing line between feeling valued and feeling slightly exploited:

> I think sometimes other professionals offload on to us sometimes, they leave some of their responsibilities on our doorstep and walk away. What I mean is, they refer a child who has whatever problem, into ... nursery, knowing that once they come, they will be observed and any problems that arise will be looked upon, and therefore in a little way they are detaching themselves away from it and passing it on to other professionals, do you know what I mean? And then that child becomes more of our responsibility and less of their responsibility and I think that often happens. You know, you feel as if you have got this child and initially there is a lot of input from the other professionals and then within a month or so you don't hear from them, and they just presume that the child is quite happy and getting on with everything at the nursery.
>
> (Nursery nurse)

We may in fact posit several possible alternative interpretations of the behaviour of these 'other professionals'. Interview data suggest that they trusted their fellow professional to take the initiative in contacting them if any aspect of the child's health or behaviour caused concern. Since not all children for whom health visitors or social workers sought nursery places were formally registered as 'at risk', there might have been no reason for them to continue to monitor the child's progress on nursery premises. Again, perhaps they were monitoring that progress through home visits and feeling well satisfied that the child was now thriving. They might have been extremely pleased with the child's development, gratefully attributing the improvement to the benign influence of the nursery. The problem, from the perspective of promoting multiprofessional working, was that the reason for discontinuing nursery visits had not been communicated to the nursery nurse. With better communication, she might have felt valued, rather than simply taken for granted.

Several other interviewees raised issues about not feeling sufficiently or consistently valued for their professional contribution:

> They don't always appreciate how much in-depth knowledge we have of the family. It's quite often, with these 'cause for concern' families, that we have been working with them for years until there is a crisis that needs a referral. The social workers step in at crisis point and I don't think they always appreciate the amount of information we do have.
>
> (Health visitor)

> The nursery nurse, I think, is underrated for observation skills: you know, we are the first line, and we are often there when the other professionals aren't there.
>
> (Nursery nurse/outreach worker)

> I think sometimes social workers and health visitors do sometimes feel as if – how can I put it? – as if they could tell us a lot, if you know what I mean, they

have bundles and bundles of experience and information, and they often think that nursery nurses are quite young and have just come into the job and they don't think that we have had 10, 15 years' experience and have a lot under our belts as well – but I don't think that happens very often. I think they are becoming more accepting that we are professionals as well.

(Nursery nurse)

Such sentiments are not, of course, expressed only by members of wider teams. Even in hospital teams, where the potential for observing and discussing one another's contributions to the multidisciplinary team is apparently greater than in more scattered community teams, some professionals felt that their contributions to patient care were undervalued. In Chapter 12, Pearson and Spencer report similar feelings among auxiliaries and receptionists in primary health care teams.

Discussion

The chosen focus of this chapter – namely the common ground between professionals and the processes of communication and everyday contact with other professions – has inevitably left some other aspects of multiprofessional working out of focus. A different study might have concentrated on the high points of multiprofessional working in special education or in child protection, the days when the team of experts all meet for a child's annual review, or for a case conference, strategy meeting, care team meeting or even court appearances. Instead, by choosing to access information about these events primarily through interview rather than through observation, and indeed through an interview format which invited participants to start by describing their everyday role, and only moved on to clarification of multiprofessional aspects when the participant mentioned them, this project sought to uncover patterns of daily work. In order to explore what it means for individual professionals engaged in their everyday routines to be part of the wider team, the interview began with those everyday routines, rather than the intense experience of teamwork on the days when they meet formally as a multiprofessional team. It therefore raised questions about the relationship between the following:

- everyday work, in which the professionals interviewed were *acting* uniprofessionally, within the boundaries of their own competence and role, but demonstrated that they were often *thinking* multiprofessionally about questions which they intended to raise with colleagues from different professions, and seeking opportunities for informal contact with those colleagues; and
- the more intense, but relatively infrequent experience of formal team meetings and decision-making processes.

Other researchers (Engstrœm, 1986; Sands *et al.*, 1990; Tisdall, 1994; Hallett, 1995) have made more detailed studies of such formal teams in action. Birchall and Hallett (1995) and Bass (1995) have commented on the high level of anxiety experienced by professionals working on child protection cases, and the data collected in this project confirmed that anxiety increased when a court appearance was imminent. Bass (1995) has discussed the value of specialist child protection advisers in the health visiting service. In this study, too, a senior health visitor was frequently mentioned as a source of support, appreciated not only by health visitors, but also by social workers and nursery nurses in the wider team. Several other instances of interprofessional support at these crisis points were cited. Equally apparent was the importance placed by anxious professionals on informal contacts outside the formal team forum, both for gathering information on which to base professional judgements and for building a sense of being a member of a team, a feeling which appeared to oil the wheels of formal teamwork when meetings did take place for statutory purposes.

Alternatively, the spotlight might have been placed on interprofessional tensions and disagreements. Inevitably, a range of these figured in the data across the whole project, from misunderstandings to the occasional blazing row. While a few of these conflicts appeared to be blatantly destructive to interprofessional working, most might be classed as, in the words of a senior teacher in the special school, 'productive disharmony'. Buckenham and McGrath (1983) have drawn attention to the danger, in hospital settings, of loyalty to the team exceeding commitment to the patient. In the wider teams studied in the present project this did not appear to be a problem. The professionals interviewed for this project were generally aware of the contributions of other professionals to the welfare of their clients, patients or pupils. They acknowledged those contributions and were prepared to work flexibly in the interests of clients, and they saw the need to collaborate and share information – but they did not necessarily feel under pressure to agree with colleagues' assessments of shared clients' needs. Mutual respect did not preclude clashes of opinion over programmes of support for clients. Øvretveit (1995) describes the need in teams for a 'circle of creative conflict', with a culture of respect and trust which allows differences of opinion and conflict to be aired and resolved, and where differences energize the team, as opposed to the vicious circle based on a culture of mistrust and suspicion, where differences become destructive. Creating a team climate in which conflict can be aired and serious differences of opinion can be resolved through open debate is not easy if the team is convened formally, perhaps only once a month or, in the case of school reviews, only a few times a year. The quality of the team climate on the occasions when it does meet formally clearly depends considerably on the everyday working relationships of the individual members of the team.

Finally, although these wider teams are much more varied and diffuse than most primary health care teams discussed elsewhere in this book, many of the findings may be of relevance to members of those teams, as developments in community care bring them into working relationships with an ever-widening array of other professional and paraprofessional workers. If staff are too numerous, too heterogeneous and too scattered to be incorporated into a formally managed multiprofessional team, or even to be invited to teambuilding events, perhaps we need not despair. The ability of staff to find their own ways of working together, to build relationships and to find common ground should not be underestimated.

Editors' summary

In this chapter, Edward has presented quite a different notion of team-working in primary health care, focusing on the complex relationships between professionals working in two community contexts – a special needs school and a community nursery. She has explored the common ground in professionals' approaches to their work, concluding that they demonstrate overlapping approaches in flexible working, in accessibility (to clients and to one another) and in valuing the contributions of other professionals. She has concluded that, in everyday work, professionals are often *acting* uni-professionally whilst *thinking* multiprofessionally. More infrequently, they are involved in formal team meetings and interdisciplinary decision-making processes. Since we do not spend all our time in team meetings or with the whole spectrum of our colleagues, these ideas have an important role in filling the gaps in our thinking about teamwork in primary care.

References

Bass A (1995) Supporting health visitors in child protection. *Health Visitor* 68, 410–11.

Belbin M (1993) *Team Roles at Work.* Butterworth-Heinemann, Oxford.

Birchall E and Hallett C (1995) Working together in child protection. *Health Visitor* 68, 406–9.

Buckenham JE and McGrath G (1983) *The Social Reality of Nursing.* ADIS Health Science Press, Sydney.

Department of Health (1989) *The Children Act 1989.* HMSO, London.

Department of Health (1993) *The Children Act Report 1992.* HMSO, London.

Engstrœm B (1986) Communication and decision-making in a study of a multi-disciplinary team conference with the registered nurse as conference chairman. *International Journal of Nursing Studies* 23, 299–314.

Eraut M (1994) *Developing Professional Knowledge and Competence.* Falmer, London.

Hallett C (1995) *Interagency Coordination in Child Protection.* HMSO, London.

Home Office Department of Health, Department of Education and Science and the Welsh Office (1991) *Working Together Under the Children Act: A Guide to Arrangements for Interagency Cooperation for the Protection of Children.* HMSO, London.

Nason F (1983) Diagnosing the hospital team. *Social Work in Health Care* 9, 25–45.

Øvretveit J (1993) *Coordinating Community Care: Multidisciplinary Teams and Care Management*. Open University Press, Buckingham.

Øvretveit J (1995) Team decision-making. *Journal of Interprofessional Care* 9, 41–51.

Reed J and Procter S (eds) (1995) *Practitioner Research in Health Care*. Chapman & Hall, London.

Ringelmann M (1913) Recherches sur les moteurs animés: travail de l'homme. *Annales de l'Institut National Agronomique Series 2*, 12, 1–40.

Rowe J, Wing J and Peters L (1995) Working with vulnerable families: the impact on health visitor workloads. *Health Visitor* 68, 232–5.

Sands RG, Staford J and McClelland M (1990) I beg to differ: conflict in the interdisciplinary team. *Social Work in Health Care* 14, 55–72.

Strauss A, Schatzmann L, Ehrlich D, Bucher R and Sabshin M (1963) The hospital and its negotiated order. Reprinted in Salaman G and Thompson K, *People and Organizations*, pp. 303–20. Longman, London.

Tisdall EKM (1994) *Effective Transitional Planning for Young Disabled People Leaving School*. Paper presented at the Scottish Educational Research Association Conference, St Andrews, 1994.

Webb C (1987) The nurse as advocate: professionalism revisited. *Nursing Times* 83, 39–41.

West MA and Poulton BC (1997) Primary health care teams: a failure of function. *Journal of Interprofessional Care*, in press.

Acknowledgements

I wish to thank all of the professionals who participated in the research, my colleagues at the University of Northumbria – Professor Colin Biott, Helen Close, Margaret Moran and Professor Sue Procter – and Dr Julie Allan, University of Stirling.

5

Teamcare Valleys – a multifaceted approach to teambuilding in primary health care

Ros Bryar

Introduction

In recent years, as discussed in other chapters of this book, there has been increasing concern about standards of primary health care provision. This concern has focused on problems in inner cities, but other areas, such as the South Wales Valleys which have experienced long-term economic decline through the rundown of traditional industries such as coalmining and metal-works, appear to experience similar problems (Lorentzon et al., 1994). In such areas the pressures on primary health care staff are enormous, as members of the community experience the cumulative effects of unemployment, low incomes and deprivation on their health. As Lorentzon et al. (1994, p. 1) comment: 'General practitioners and other primary health care professionals find themselves at the sharp end of seeking to deal with increasing health and social need, often finding the latter overwhelming.'

Teambuilding has long been advocated as a means of both improving the outcomes of care and providing support mechanisms for those working in primary health care. While the evidence for the effectiveness of teamwork in these two areas is still being accumulated, personal experience and anecdotal evidence from members of both functioning and non-functioning primary health care teams (PHCTs) suggest that teams of primary health care practitioners who are working effectively together can provide a different type of service to communities and gain considerable personal support from the team environment.

In Wales, the South Wales Valleys are an area of significant deprivation. In 1988, the University of Wales College of Medicine was given the opportunity to establish a primary health care development project in the Valleys. The project was entitled Teamcare Valleys (TCV), reflecting the widely held view in primary health care that teams contribute to better care, and also indicating that teams themselves need care if they are to be maintained and developed. TCV was a 3-year, multidisciplinary project which utilised a multifaceted approach to supporting the development of primary health care. The aim of this chapter is to provide a description of some aspects of the work of TCV which contributed to the development and understanding of teamwork in primary health care.

Context of the work of TCV

As with all of the projects described in this collection, the work of TCV needs to be located in both place and time: 'Perhaps the main point to remember is that, in the face of so many problems, it is a tribute to the tenacity of the Valley communities that so many people believe that remedies can, and should, be found' (Morgan and Price, 1992, pp. 37–8). The South Wales Valleys is an area consisting of 26 valleys, bounded to the north by the Heads of the Valleys road and the Brecon Beacons and to the south by the M4 motorway and the coastal belt. The area extends from Pontypool in the east to Crosshands in the west, and covers most of the area of the former South Wales coalfield. The population is approximately 700 000, which is equivalent to the population of a city such as Manchester (Bryar and Bytheway, 1996). There are several towns in the Valleys, but the major population centres of Cardiff, Bridgend and Swansea are located to the south of the area.

The Valleys have experienced long-term decline in employment since the 1920s, although the popular view is still that of an area steeped in the traditions of mining communities. While many of the traditions and much of the cohesiveness may still exist, the reality of many people's lives is bleak.

> More significant is the extraordinary level of dependency. Less than half of the people of working age are actually in full-time employment, the rest being unemployed, permanently sick or disabled, caring for homes and families, prematurely retired or working only part-time. Furthermore, 60% of the districts have a higher than national average of elderly people.
>
> (Morgan and Price, 1992, p. 28)

The problems that had become endemic in the area led Peter Walker, then Secretary of State for Wales, to launch *The Valleys – A Programme for the People* (Welsh Office, 1988). This was an extensive initiative aimed at halting decline through a range of activities, including the generation of new jobs, upgrading of housing, improvement of the environment, encouragement of the arts and music, implementation of community development activities and undertaking of health projects, including the upgrading of some hospitals. TCV was one of the health projects, funded at a cost of £3 million by the Welsh Office, within this wider political and social programme. The initial statements about TCV indicate the emphasis that was placed on the development of teamwork by instigators of the project:

> The Welsh Office will take a number of new initiatives designed to support the development of primary health care services for Valleys communities. The intention will be to extend vocational training for health professionals working in the Valleys and to provide a more direct role for the University of Wales College of Medicine. Measures to support improved teamwork in the primary care field will also be devised.
>
> (Welsh Office, 1988, p. 31)

TCV was therefore a project instigated by political leaders, rather than by practitioners, and it formed part of a wider political initiative with a remit far beyond the aims of supporting the development and provision of primary health care services. As suggested by the above quotation, the focus of the project was on the health care practitioners. It was anticipated that if support and development activities were provided for primary health care practitioners this would result in an improved primary health care service for the community.

TCV was launched in 1990 and concluded in August 1993. Within the Valleys area there are approximately 156 general practices (during the 3 years of the project there were a number of mergers and separations) with whom TCV sought to work. TCV was assigned by its Steering Group to work with the 'traditional' PHCT, consisting of general practitioners, practice management staff, practice nurses and the attached community nurses, midwives, health visitors and psychiatric nurses. In total it was estimated that there were 2000 of these primary care practitioners in the area. In addition, TCV sought to establish working relationships with the local health authorities. In 1990, there were five health authorities and five Family Health Service Authorities (FHSAs) in the Valleys. Sections of these 10 authorities fell within the boundaries of the Valleys, but none had its total population within the area. The year 1990 was a significant one in that it saw the publication of the new GP Contract, the first since 1966, which, with the implementation of the contract culture in the NHS from 1991 onwards, heralded enormous changes in the structures, management and working practices of the NHS in general, and primary health care in particular (see Chapter 3). TCV aimed to support the development of primary health care, and the launch of a project at a time of organisational uncertainty in the NHS hampered its work. For example, nurse managers commented towards the end of the 3 years that they felt they had not had the time to make full use of the resource provided by TCV, because of the need to focus their energies on the issues of organisational change, including the establishment of NHS Trusts.

A multidisciplinary unit

TCV was created as an academic unit within the University of Wales College of Medicine. It had a full-time staff consisting of a director, administrator, project board co-ordinators and 'long-term clinical fellows'. In addition, it funded a number of short-term appointments, to TCV, of health care practitioners working in the Valleys (Wallace, 1993). These practitioners were seconded to TCV for varying lengths of time in order to undertake individual projects that were concerned with their practice, and were referred to as 'short-term clinical fellows'. A multidisciplinary group of people drawn from general practice, nursing, health visiting, practice management, health promotion, social science research, community midwifery, community psychiatric nursing, nurse education and continuing medical education, with an administrator and secretaries, made up the group of 53 people who were employed during the 3 years by TCV. The composition of TCV therefore reflected the groups of staff working in primary health care. As a result of working together on a range of projects, everyone who worked at TCV learned a great deal about the work of different professional groups. In the activities undertaken we were able to demonstrate the synergistic effects of teamwork or the 'added value' achieved through combining our expertise in the development of educational courses, research projects and support activities in practices.

Pendleton (1995) advocates the establishment of a multidisciplinary professional development consultancy service in primary health care, which would address both the individual needs of practitioners and the organisational needs of practices and other primary care organisations. TCV provides evidence of the value of such a multifaceted approach which seeks to support and influence change through a range of different activities at the various levels. The aim of TCV was to help to develop PHC in the Valleys area as the mission statement identifies:

> As a unit of the University of Wales College of Medicine, Teamcare Valleys will, in collaboration and dialogue with authorities and other agencies, support the development of primary health care services for the Valleys communities, by stimulating interest and engagement amongst those involved in primary health care, pioneering a blend of support and advice for primary health care practitioners with continuing education and training, and assisting in primary health care team development.
>
> (Teamcare Valleys, 1993, p. 5)

In order to fulfil these aims, the work of the project was grouped into four main areas:

- communication;
- education and training;
- field projects;
- practical support and advice.

Within each of these areas a range of projects was undertaken. For example, a total of 31 field projects and 25 education and training projects were initiated, of which 26 and 21 projects, respectively, were completed. All of the projects undertaken had to fulfil a number of criteria before they could be initiated, including the requirement that each project promoted 'the positive benefits of multi- and interdisciplinary team working in primary care (for the community and practitioners alike) through training and other practical measures' (Teamcare Valleys, 1993, p. 7). Each of the projects made a significant contribution to the work of TCV, and many projects reinforced one another. For example, PHC practitioners who attended outreach events concerning the project (Roadshows) subsequently became short-term clinical fellows or encouraged their team members to attend a TCV course. In the following sections of this chapter a description of one project from each of the main programme areas is provided. The projects chosen demonstrate in particular the contribution of TCV to the development of teamwork. For those seeking further information about the work of TCV, the final Overview Report (Teamcare Valleys, 1993) provides a list of all TCV publications, and Bryar and Bytheway (1996) have edited a collection of reports on 23 projects undertaken by TCV.

Communication

One of the most important tasks was to develop methods of communicating with the practices and other organisations involved in primary health care, to disseminate examples of good practice, to reduce the isolation of practitioners, and to ensure that people were informed about the activities being undertaken by TCV. As described above, the geographical terrain of the Valleys militates against easy communication between health care practitioners and between PHCTs, leading to a feeling of isolation among practitioners. This isolation was reinforced by the difficulties of travelling in an area consisting of steep-sided valleys, and the small size of many teams, which meant that individual practitioners might feel isolated from members of their own professional group. The isolation of practitioners was also reinforced by the lack of communication between teams in the area. This not only reduced opportunities for support, but also limited the diffusion of good practice. In addition, teamwork in practices was not well developed, contributing further to the isolation of practitioners. In the early days of TCV the clinical fellows conducted a needs assessment by visiting as many practices as possible within the area. As part of this they undertook a classification of teamwork in the practices based on discussions with practice team members. Approximately 90 per cent of the practices were visited, and in 33 per cent of these it was estimated that teamwork was poor. (Bytheway, 1991).

In an effort to encourage dissemination of information and to aid networking, support and teamworking on a wider scale between members of

PHTCs, a range of publications were produced by TCV. These included discussion papers, project reports and the quarterly newsletter *ReValley*. Discussion papers were produced by members of TCV and by people working with TCV on topics relating to clinical practice, research and education, and they included papers on behavioural work with children (Pritchard and Bytheway, 1992), interpreting the drop-out of GPs from distance-learning courses (Middleton *et al.*, 1992), continuing medication (Venn, 1991) and action research (English, 1991). The papers were produced and distributed while each project continued, and provided a means of ensuring that the projects were relevant and enabled a wide range of people to contribute to their development. Each of the papers contained a number of questions, and readers were asked to return their responses to these questions. The responses contributed to the further development of projects, e.g. the recruitment of a practice (Thomas, 1993), or to a new discussion paper (English, 1992).

It was a requirement that each project should be written up when it ended, and that a project report should be produced. These reports were circulated to the practices involved in the project and to other interested individuals. Copies of the reports were also sent out to local medical, postgraduate and nursing libraries in the area. Each report contained suggestions for further activities, as well as a description of the project. Some projects also produced guidelines on, for example, running sleep clinics (Hitch, 1993) or introducing computers in general practice (English, 1993).

A quarterly newsletter, entitled *ReValley*, was distributed to the practices and other organisations in the area. *ReValley* aimed to be 'informative, educational and supportive' (Teamcare Valleys, 1991) and contained information about TCV activities, initiatives in practices, educational activities, including study days and courses, as well as information about other local resources. The newsletter was edited by Julie Slater, a clinical fellow, for the first year, and then, as the work on her project on stress in PHCTs expanded, it was taken over by Bill Bytheway, Senior Lecturer in Social Science. Practitioners contributed short articles on innovations in practice, e.g. a breast care support group initiated by district nurses and a coronary support group run by a health visitor. Clinical fellows reported on the progress of their projects, e.g. on asthma in children and setting up GP diabetic clinics. New courses were advertised, e.g. 'Ophthalmology for General Practitioners', and information was provided about the progress of support groups such as the Practice Managers' Support Group initiated by TCV. Photographs were used to show people activities such as the Roadshows and Conference. In a number of issues the back page was used to ask readers for specific information, e.g. on audit services in the area and the number and content of asthma clinics. Individuals from organisations supporting the work of PHCTs in the area provided articles describing their work, e.g. as a health promotion officer or practice nurse facilitator.

ReValley thus enabled the distribution of information on a regular basis to all of the practices in the Valleys, as well as to other organisations associated with primary health care. It made possible the sharing of information across practice and other administrative boundaries over a wide geographical area, and it also gave practitioners the opportunity to prepare a short article and thus to develop confidence in writing for publication.

Education

One means of developing teamwork is through education. While it may be argued that teamwork in primary health care would be best achieved through joint initial education of health care practitioners, continuing education for qualified practitioners can achieve a great deal. Educational courses are generally held in educational centres, but TCV made the decision early on that courses should be held as near as possible to the area where the practitioners worked (mirroring the philosophy that primary care services for the community should be provided as close as possible to the area where people live and work). The educational centres serving the Valleys are located in the major cities and towns south of the area, and travel to these centres can be fairly time-consuming, making it difficult for practitioners to attend courses.

Community and public health in the Valleys

As one means of overcoming this problem, TCV developed a number of distance-learning courses and a 9-month course entitled 'Community and Public Health in the Valleys', which combined workbooks (distance learning) with study days and tutorials held in the area. The course was first proposed by David Middleton, a social scientist who joined TCV as a research officer. The course planning team consisted of the director of TCV (who had a general practice background), the lecturer in practice management and two nurses. The team was supplemented by other members of the TCV with social science, general practice and nursing backgrounds who were involved in study days, tutorials and marking coursework. Thus the course illustrates the multidisciplinary work of TCV – this team had to resolve its own differences of opinion, e.g. with regard to educational methods and marking standards, which were influenced by the different backgrounds of the team members involved.

The course aimed to develop participants' understanding of the social, economic and cultural influences on health in the area through exploration of underlying theory, local statistics and examination of an issue of relevance to their own practice. The course also sought to develop participants' confidence as self-directed adult learners, enabling them to pursue further self-directed study in the future. Another objective of the course was to help participants to gain a greater understanding of the roles of the different people and organisations involved in primary health care through participation in the course.

The second underlying principle of the course is that education for people in primary health care should be provided in a multidisciplinary setting. Course members will gain an increased understanding of the roles of different people through undertaking the course together, enabling them to work more constructively in their own primary health care teams.

(Slater, 1993, p. 2)

A total of 34 people enrolled on the course, including district nurses, GPs, practice nurses, specialist nurses, people employed in FHSAs and community health councils and a health visitor. The course was given postgraduate education allowance (PGEA) approval, and was also validated by the Welsh National Board (WNB) so that nurses who satisfactorily completed the course gained a diploma credit towards the WNB Diploma in Professional Practice. The course members attended three workshop days held in different venues across the Valleys. They were divided into a number of multidisciplinary tutorial groups according to geographical location, and met on four occasions for group tutorials in a convenient practice which had a suitable room to accommodate them. Each tutorial group was facilitated by two members of staff from TCV, the members of each pair having different professional expertise, e.g. a GP and a nurse worked together, and a GP and a social scientist. The course was evaluated in a number of ways, including pre- and post-module knowledge assessments, workshop evaluations, tutorial discussions and written evaluations.

The evaluation of the course concluded that its multidisciplinary nature was one of its greatest successes. On the first day it was apparent that some course members found it difficult to express their views in a mixed group, but over the 9 months all of them developed greater confidence through attending the tutorials and workshops. As one GP commented: 'I've found it refreshing to be argued with by nurses who usually seem to be convinced that they can't tell doctors anything about medicine' (Slater, 1993, p. 14). A district nurse commented: 'TCV's inter-disciplinary approach is a refreshing change – let's all work together' (Slater, 1993, p. 14).

The course thus helped individuals to gain a greater understanding of the roles of other members of the PHCT with practitioners (in most cases) with whom they were not working on a day-to-day basis. In the educational environment of the workshop and the tutorial they were able to challenge and test colleagues in ways that they might not have found possible within their own teams. Having had this opportunity, they might then be able to work in different ways with members of their own PHCTs.

Field projects

These projects were undertaken mainly by both long- and short-term clinical fellows, with the support of members of TCV, practitioners and other individuals in other local organisations, including schools, the university and

FHSAs. Field projects contributed to the development of primary health care through investigation of an issue of concern to primary care practitioners and others, the development of the individual through the acquisition of research skills in a supportive environment and the development of team-work.

Teamwork was developed in a number of ways. Individual projects often arose from the suggestions of a number of people either in one practice team or in a number of practices who shared the same concerns. A study of the educational needs of practice nurses arose as a result of concern in a number of practices about this issue (Davies, 1993). This project was teamed with another TCV project which was investigating the setting up of diabetic clinics in the same practices (Wallis, 1993). The majority of the projects were undertaken by one person, but all involved other practitioners to a greater or lesser extent during the course of the project. For example, in a study of standard setting in one practice, the clinical fellow acted as the facilitator for a group that included nurses, a health visitor, a GP and a receptionist (Gill, 1992). In another study the GP (who was appointed as a short-term clinical fellow) and a practice nurse conducted a project designed to test different educational methods (Thapar, 1993). In the final report of this project, the benefits of the project to team cohesiveness were identified:

> More teamwork resulted from group education being done with the practice nurse, and from receptionists being involved in questionnaire distribution and collection – they were very curious about the results! . . . Improved morale – the practice team feels 'progressive' and have valued positive patient feedback.
>
> (Thapar, 1993, p. 16)

Other projects were undertaken by pairs of individuals or small teams. A group of four midwives was concerned to understand the needs of women in their patch prior to the introduction of change (Marx *et al.*, 1993), and were appointed as a team. Different team members were responsible for the different stages of the survey that they undertook. One member of the team took on the overall co-ordinating role for the project. Team members felt that they had gained individually from conducting the project. They had gained practical experience in undertaking a project, and this also initiated active reflective practice in the team. Discussion of and reflection on the responses to the questionnaires led to a greater appreciation amongst the team of one another's strengths and weaknesses (Marx, 1996). Another team consisted of eight community psychiatric nurses, some of whom were appointed as a team with a research nurse to a short-term clinical fellow's post, and undertook a study of definitions of depression (Proctor *et al.*, 1996). This group also found that working on the project revealed hidden talents: 'Working as a group helped to further build relationships, and respect for individuals grew as hidden talents and knowledge emerged' (Proctor *et al.*, 1996). This team also found that they needed a project co-ordinator, as the demands of busy caseloads often drew people away from project work. This suggests that in PHCT practice the appointment of a co-ordinator for a practice initiative might lead to greater success in carrying through projects. Although working as a team presented additional stresses, the pairs of individuals and the team valued the support provided by working together, and a number of the full-time clinical fellows considered that if they had undertaken a team project they would not have felt so isolated in the new role of 'researcher' (Pritchard, 1996).

Practical support and advice

Practices may experience considerable problems, including how to undertake recruitment, how to organise work between different team members, how to meet financial obligations, how to organise recall systems, and many more. To help team members with such problems, TCV set up a Practice Advisory Service (PAS). The core members included the director of TCV, the lecturer in practice management and myself, providing a resource for the teams with experience in general practice, management and nursing (Wallace, 1996). Teams in general referred themselves to the service, but in one project six practices were referred to the service by the FHSA. FHSAs had a particular relationship with practices, and TCV, as an independent agency, was able to complement the work of the FHSA by providing practice-based advice and support, as well as helping the practices to negotiate for additional resources from the FHSA.

Team meetings were held with the six practices, enabling everyone to express their views about two areas identified for attention, namely cervical cytology uptake and immunisation. Individual and joint activities took place. For example, the lecturer in practice management worked with practice management staff to organise call and recall systems. This work identified issues related to different information systems in the community services and FHSA. On the nursing side, deficits in education were identified in conjunction with the FHSA nurse advisor, and practical and theoretical input was provided. A joint study day for all team members was also held on the subject of immunisation, as conflicting advice from different team members had been identified at the initial meetings.

This project involved teamwork between TCV and one FHSA, as well as teamwork between members of the staff of TCV and a number of practices, and between individuals in the practices. Links were also made between a number of the practices. Workload, the demands of different information systems, inadequate resources or inadequate use of resources were found to hamper these practices in their work. By being brought together, individuals realised where there was an overlap of information, and in many cases were able to generate their own solutions. Through this process they developed better teamworking.

Conclusions

This chapter provides an overview of the work of Teamcare Valleys. Teamwork and the development of teamwork formed a major strand woven through all of the Teamcare Valleys projects, but examples have been given here of some areas in which team development was a more explicit rather than implicit element. Some of the conclusions which may be drawn from the work of Teamcare Valley are as follows:

- PHCTs benefit from the multifaceted support provided by a unit such as Teamcare Valleys. Development and change in primary care may be more readily achieved through the provision of support which is multidisciplinary, flexible, independent and able to respond to the full range of needs of practices. In short, PHCTs need 'care'.
- Teamcare Valleys may be unique among PHCT development projects in the extent to which it was associated with a political rather than a primary health care initiative. However, all primary care initiatives need to be mindful of the political context in which they are established and in which they seek to achieve their outcomes.
- The multidisciplinary staffing of Teamcare Valleys was vital in enabling us to understand and respond to the different needs of the various team members. It also resulted in considerable learning by Teamcare Valleys staff about the roles of different primary care practitioners.
- Teamcare Valleys was able to work at different levels and on a wide range of activities with individuals, practices and other organisations, e.g. FHSAs and community units. This could be described as an holistic approach to primary care development, and it had the potential to achieve greater change than working at only one level.
- The isolation of primary health care practitioners was reinforced in this case by geography, but is an issue in many primary care settings, and can be reduced by better information distribution, education and other means. The isolation of practitioners and practices may be one of the most important features limiting the development of primary health care practice.
- Multidisciplinary education enables individuals to work with and challenge people in different professional groups and may be particularly effective in aiding teamwork when individuals are able to undertake courses with other teams.
- Teamcare Valleys was able to provide a range of educational activities run by multidisciplinary groups role modelling teamwork in the process.
- Individual project work by PHCT members was found to stimulate teamwork and to develop a feeling of enhanced worth in the practices.
- Change in practice, including the development of teamwork, was found to occur more readily when education was combined with practical support and advice in the practice setting, such as that provided by the Practice Advisory Service.

Editors' summary _____

Bryar's chapter has offered an overview of the work of Teamcare Valleys, perhaps one of the most exciting initiatives in primary care development to emerge in the early 1990s. She has outlined the political nature of the project, and its sense of being part of a far wider initiative aimed at regenerating the life of the Welsh Valleys. She has described the very wide range of projects undertaken by the team in the areas of communication, education and training, field projects and practical support and advice. However, Teamcare Valleys ceased to be funded in 1993. Although the impact of the project on multidisciplinary working appears to have been considerable, Bryar has also described the difficulties encountered by the team in the face of extensive organisational change and uncertainty. Very often, primary care development at all levels is caught up within political agendas, and must respond to these. They will not always be so explicit. Political agendas change, and there is no guarantee of long-term funding. Impact in areas such as team development must therefore be achieved rapidly, and maintained with minimal resources.

References

Bryar R and Bytheway B (1996) *Changing Primary Health Care. The Teamcare Valleys Experience*. Blackwell Science, Oxford.

Bytheway B (1991) *Primary Health Care Needs*. Teamcare Valleys Discussion Paper No. 8. Teamcare Valleys, Welsh Office, Cardiff.

Davies K (1993) *Review of the Training Needs of Practice Nurses in Diabetes Health Care in the Rhondda Health Unit*. Teamcare Valleys Report. Teamcare Valleys, Welsh Office, Cardiff.

English P (1991) *Action Research and Primary Care*. Teamcare Valleys Discussion Paper No. 5. Teamcare Valleys, Welsh Office, Cardiff.

English P (1992) *Responses to Discussion Paper No. 5*. Teamcare Valleys Discussion Paper No. 11. Teamcare Valleys, Welsh Office, Cardiff.

English P (1993) *An Introduction to Computers in Primary Health Care*. Teamcare Valleys Report. Teamcare Valleys, Welsh Office, Cardiff.

Gill J (1992) *Setting Multidisciplinary Standards of Care*. Teamcare Valleys Report. Teamcare Valleys, Welsh Office, Cardiff.

Hitch A (1993) *Distance Learning Pack for Health Professionals. Working With Families in the Community – Helping Children Under Five Years of Age to Develop Good Sleeping Patterns*. Teamcare Valleys Report. Teamcare Valleys, Welsh Office, Cardiff.

Lorentzon M, Jarman B and Bajekal M (1994) *Report of the Inner City Task Force of the Royal College of General Practitioners*. Occasional Paper No. 66. Royal College of General Practitioners, London.

Marx R (1996) Providing continuity of care by community midwives. In Bryar R and Bytheway B (eds) *Changing Primary Health Care. The Teamcare Valleys Experience*, pp. 181–91. Blackwell Science, Oxford.

Marx R, Isaac G, Jones A and Rowlands M (1993) *Continuity of Care From Community Midwives: A Study into the Satisfaction and Future Needs of Women in the Amman Valley Area*. Teamcare Valleys Report. Teamcare Valleys, Welsh Office, Cardiff.

Middleton D, Edwards P and Houston H (1992) *I've Started so I'll Finish: GPs and Drop-Out Rates from Distance Learning Packages*. Teamcare Valleys Discussion Paper No. 12. Teamcare Valleys, Welsh Office, Cardiff.

Morgan K and Price A (1992) *Re-Building our Communities. A New Agenda for the Valleys*. Department of City and Regional Planning, University of Wales College of Cardiff, Cardiff.

Pendleton D (1995) Professional development in general practice: problems, puzzles and paradigms. *British Journal of General Practice* 45, 377–81.

Pritchard P and Bytheway B (1992) *Behavioural Work in the Community with Pre-School Children*. Teamcare Valleys Discussion Paper No. 13. Teamcare Valleys, Welsh Office, Cardiff.

Pritchard R (1996) Feeling uneasy about research. In Bryar R and Bytheway B (eds) *Changing Primary Health Care. The Teamcare Valleys Experience*, pp. 119–27. Blackwell Science, Oxford.

Proctor H, Davies P and Lewis P (1996) Understanding depression in the community. In Bryar R and Bytheway B (eds) *Changing Primary Health Care. The Teamcare Valleys Experience*, pp. 167–76. Blackwell Science, Oxford.

Slater J (1993) *Community and Public Health in the Valleys*. Evaluation Report. Teamcare Valleys, Welsh Office, Cardiff.

Teamcare Valleys (1991) *ReValley*. The Newsletter of Teamcare Valleys. No. 1, Spring 1991. Welsh Office, Cardiff.

Teamcare Valleys (1993) *University of Wales College of Medicine Teamcare Valleys 1990–1993*. Overview Report. Teamcare Valleys, Welsh Office, Cardiff.

Thapar A (1993) *Patient Education in Asthma. A Comparison Between Small Group Education and Individual Counselling*. Teamcare Valleys Report. Teamcare Valleys, Welsh Office, Cardiff.

Thomas A (1993) *'That's What We're There For ... the Patients.' A Qualitative Study of Perceived Health Need*. Teamcare Valleys Report. Teamcare Valleys, Welsh Office, Cardiff.

Venn C (1991) *Continuing Medication in the Community – Is It a Problem?* Teamcare Valleys Discussion Paper No. 7. Teamcare Valleys, Welsh Office, Cardiff.

Wallace B (1993) The Teamcare Valleys initiative. *Health and Social Care in the Community* 1, 61–4.

Wallace B (1996) Helping to resolve problems in the development of practices. In Bryar R and Bytheway B (eds) *Changing Primary Health Care. The Teamcare Valleys Experience*, pp. 24–32. Blackwell Science, Oxford.

Wallis D (1993) *The Teamcare Valleys Diabetic Mini-Clinics Project. Final Report*. Teamcare Valleys Report. Teamcare Valleys, Welsh Office, Cardiff.

Welsh Office (1988) *The Valleys – A Programme for the People*. Welsh Office, Cardiff.

6

Promoting teamwork through health promotion

Susan Gooding

Introduction

This chapter describes the impact, effectiveness and development of an ongoing multidisciplinary, multiprofessional, multi-agency team development programme for primary health care teams (PHCTs) in England. The initiative, known as the Multidisciplinary Primary Health Care Team Workshop (MDTW) programme, has been developed by the Health Education Authority (HEA) since 1987.

The major component of the programme is the provision of a series of guided learning events for PHCTs organised by Local Organising Teams (LOTs). The learning events are designed to provide the opportunity for those working in primary health care to reflect on their current health promotion and disease prevention practices and subsequently to develop strategies to enhance their activities. The health promotion planning and problem-solving model is the vehicle for encouraging and developing teamwork skills between members of the group of primary health care workers.

Local Organising Teams consist of representatives from family health services authorities, community trusts, health commissions, health authorities, general practice, universities or postgraduate training offices and, increasingly, from social services and voluntary agencies. There are currently 70 LOTs throughout England.

Evaluation of the MDTW programme for both PHCTs and LOTs, and of subsequent follow-up and support for the programme, indicates that it is an effective mechanism for developing and enhancing the work that the PHCT undertakes in the area of health promotion and disease prevention. Those participating in the programme also report that it has enhanced communication, teamwork and practice organisation. More than 10 per cent of practices in England have taken part in the programme.

Origins of the programme

The importance of teamwork has been recognised in a number of key reports, including the Harding (Department of Health and Social Security, 1981), Acheson (London Health Planning Consortium, in Acheson, 1981) and Cumberlege Reports (Department of Health and Social Security, 1986). Teamworking is not an easy option for primary health care teams. Potential barriers include contractual and professional divisions between, for example, general practitioners (GPs), district nurses, health visitors and other team members; differences in management structures and account- ability (GPs are independent contractors, and practice nurses, practice man- agers and administrative and support staff are employed by the GP, while community nurses, dietitians, social workers and physiotherapists are usu- ally employed by other health care agencies); team members may find their loyalty divided between the general practitioner and their managers; team members may work from different premises and attached staff may work with a number of practices; where roles overlap distrust and suspicion can be generated; the diverse professionals and disciplines forming a PHCT have different learning styles and educational experiences, their training has varied in length and has required different learning styles and educational experiences, and inevitably among the members of the PHCT there are dif- ferent levels of commitment to a philosophy of teamworking.

Successful health promotion and disease prevention require contributions from a diverse range of individuals – many of whom have no formal training in the specialism – working in a variety of settings. A team approach to health promotion and disease prevention provides the opportunity for a group of people to combine their skills, knowledge and experience to offer a sensitive, effective, creative service to their practice population. Each member of the PHCT brings to health promotion something different, essential and unique. Individual contributions in health promotion can be identifiable.

From very small beginnings the MDTW programme has developed into a multifaceted network of activity across England. The programme is currently supported by 70 LOTs, who encourage PHCTs to take time out of their busy working schedules in order to develop health promotion and prevention activities which can be readily integrated with the everyday work of general practice.

Since the MDTW programme started in 1987, primary health care has experienced many changes, including the introduction of the 1990 GP Contract (Department of Health, 1989a), changes to health promotion in that contract in 1993 (National Health Service Management Executive, 1993), the

Patient's Charter (Department of Health, 1992), Caring for People (Department of Health, 1989b) and Working for Patients (Secretaries of State for Health, Wales, Northern Ireland and Scotland, 1989). The programme has been adapted to meet and support these changes. Ongoing support has been provided by the HEA National Unit for Health Promotion in Primary Care, Oxford.

The main focus in the early stages of the programme was the launching of the first distance-learning pack by the Open University, financed by the Health Education Council/Health Education Advisory, entitled 'Coronary Heart Disease – Reducing the Risk.' With the introduction of the 1990 GP Contract, much of the focus was turned to the development of health promotion clinics. When changes were introduced to the health promotion component of the Contract in 1993, PHCTs used the programme to prepare themselves for the banding system and to work towards obtaining Band 3 status. As developments in primary care have occurred, the agenda for PHCTs has changed so as to reflect them, but teamwork, health promotion and disease prevention have remained central.

The original aims of the MDTW Programme were as follows. First, it aimed to provide an opportunity for those working in primary health care to plan activities in disease prevention and health promotion, or to update ongoing activities, within the practice population and within the constraints of each individual practice – based on teamwork and co-operation with other health professionals. Secondly, the programme aimed to encourage understanding of the role and skills of each profession and discipline, and to stimulate inter-professional communication and teamwork to achieve a common goal. Thirdly, it aimed to recognise resources that are available in the community – both lay and professional – and to make the best use of these.

The specific original objectives were as follows:

- to produce a plan for reducing the risk of coronary heart disease;
- to identify barriers and ways of overcoming these;
- to recognise facilitating factors and to develop ways of incorporating these;
- to identify the scale and nature of the problem of coronary heart disease in an individual practice;
- to establish a baseline on which strategies and targets can be established;
- to identify a target population within the practice;
- to devise an evaluation and assessment procedure to measure the effectiveness of the activity.

The key focus, initially a reduction of risk in heart disease, is now at the discretion of the LOT and their colleagues in primary health care. Greater emphasis is now placed on teamworking and team development. The programme aims primarily to increase and enhance measures in accordance with the Health of the Nation targets for reduction of risk in preventable disorder and disease. It will do this by assessing the needs of the whole population of individual practices and the community in which each practice is situated. It also aims to encourage and develop teamwork and communication skills, and to recognise and develop these skills where they are already present in primary health care workers, allied individuals, groups and agencies. In addition, the programme is intended to determine the needs of others working with primary health care teams, and to encourage the involvement of others in community resources, skills and facilities. Specific examples of the aims and objectives developed by LOTs, reflecting the shift in emphasis, can be found in the *Group Facilitation Skills Toolbox* (Health Education Authority, 1994).

There are a number of key elements in the programme's philosophy which reflect the principles of adult education. The overall programme is facilitative and participative, with each individual being respected for the skills, experience (both professional and life) and knowledge he or she can offer. The programme is structured to take between 9 and 12 months to complete. It provides opportunities for information input as appropriate, but its main emphasis is on providing the maximum opportunity for PHCTs to reflect on their existing activity and to devise strategies and plans appropriate to their own particular circumstances and needs. The LOT provides support materials and other items designed to help teams to explore different ways of developing appropriate strategies for health promotion. The richness of experience, skill and knowledge among the membership of the LOT, which the PHCT can readily tap into, provides an invaluable extra resource.

The programme is designed to be participant centred and led, rather than didactic, with the emphasis placed upon the PHCTs having the opportunity to work jointly on their strategy. It is also recognised that the participating PHCTs will probably be at different stages in the development of preventive strategies and health promotion programmes. The programme provides an opportunity to work on such initiatives in a supportive, non-competitive manner.

Design of the workshop programme

The programme is described as a series of guided learning events. During the development of the programme, its strengths have been built upon and its weaknesses addressed by the National MDTW programme team and LOTs. The programme can be divided into three distinct stages: pre-workshop activities, the workshop, and post-workshop activities.

Stage 1 – pre-workshop activity

This stage commences at least 6 months prior to the workshop stage. Experience has reinforced the importance of the contracting process in these early months. Contracting is the process of clarifying expectations and reaching agreement about the various elements of the workshop programme. It underpins the whole workshop programme, and the quality of the contracting will affect the success or otherwise of the programme. The LOT contracts with the participating PHCTs, LOT members and others who are involved with the programme. As part of the contracting process, the style of facilitation is agreed on. Facilitation of PHCTs participating in the programme differs from one LOT to another. Some LOT members 'adopt' a practice and work with its members before, during and after the workshop, some leave teams on their own but offer help should it be required, whilst others provide facilitation only during the workshop, and give general support before and after the workshop.

In order to be clear about the contract for the workshop, the LOT must agree on the aims and objectives and the intended outcomes of the programme, and its main focus. For example, some LOTs make team development the subject of the workshop. Others use health promotion as the vehicle for team development. The LOT then spends some considerable time designing, planning and organising the workshop, ideally with participating PHCTs. Preparatory work for the Stage 2 workshop should include all of the members of the PHCT although, depending on the workshop model being adopted by the LOT, not all members of the PHCT may be actively engaged in the workshop. Pre-workshop activities with PHCTs may include meetings, collection of practice baseline data, or analysis of team members' roles. Further examples can be found in the *Group Facilitation Skills Toolbox* (Health Education Authority, 1994).

Stage 2 – workshop

The original workshop model advocated a 2.5-day residential workshop. This model continues to be the most popular, as it gives PHCTs a real opportunity to focus upon themselves and to build relationships. However, other models are increasingly being adopted by LOTs, often dictated by financial constraints, but also in consultation with the needs of local PHCTs. Workshops may be residential or non-residential, whole practice days away, 1/2/3 days away, a series of away days, or short workshop sessions in the practice over a period of time. The design of the workshop is intended to reflect the different learning styles of the PHCT and the notion of an 'experiential learning cycle' (Kolb, 1984). This is explained in more detail in the *Group Facilitation Skills Toolbox* (Health Education Authority, 1994). Workshops may involve one or more PHCTs at a time.

A typical PHCT workshop will include the following: plenary activities, e.g. climate-building activity, ground-rule setting, information inputs such as understanding of non-verbal communication, practice profiling or local perspectives on coronary heart disease; uniprofessional sessions; practice team activities, e.g. role analysis or health promotion planning tasks; sessions started in plenary and followed up in practice teams, e.g. team-building in the practice, managing change or action planning; and optional sessions, e.g. quizzes, relaxation exercises such as aromatherapy, swimming or walks.

During the workshop, the PHCT develop an action plan and discuss how they are going to implement the changes that they have identified. The plans should be specific, achievable and have a realistic time scale. The plans produced by the PHCTs are as varied and unique as the teams themselves. They include activities such as the setting up of a variety of clinics (e.g. for asthma, diabetes, coronary heart disease, teenage health, Well Women, men's health), improving communication through better organised practice meetings, engaging extended PHCT members, inviting speakers to practice meetings, improving message services, appointment systems, referral systems, and computer systems, developing a children's play area in reception, holding practice open days, setting up patient participation groups, setting up community development projects, improving the decoration and ambience of the practice, and development of a practice newsletter for patients.

Stage 3 – post-workshop activity

Following the workshop there are a number of issues to address, the first being the implementation of the action plan or changes discussed at the workshop. The PHCT is responsible for following through their action plan or changes discussed at the workshop. The LOT's support and careful facilitation can help to make this happen. A further issue is that of re-entry of the participants and the re-integration of the whole PHCT in those instances where all members of the team have not experienced the workshop stage. There are sometimes difficulties when part of a team that has attended a workshop goes back to work, full of enthusiasm, their relationships closer and now more familiar, excited by new ideas and new ways of working. Those who did not attend can feel excluded and, as a consequence, may appear resistant to change. PHCTs are encouraged to build into their action plans strategies to address these issues – prevention is better than cure!

Who has attended the programme?

Since 1987 over 10 per cent of practices in England have participated in the programme. This number represents a wide range of practice types, including single-handed GPs and group practices, rural and urban locations (inner city practices as well as those situated on the periphery of towns, and practices in rural settings, some serving more isolated populations). Participating practices have included both large and small ones, some with well-established relationships and others with positive links, some who work in spacious purpose-built accommodation and others who work in cramped conditions, some who make extensive use of computers and others who do not, fundholders, non-fundholders and consortia. Although each practice is unique in its circumstances, all of the practices share fundamental characteristics, which means that they can all address the same planning task in order to develop strategies appropriate to their own specific circumstances.

Practice development is, of course, related to many factors, including the extent to which multidisciplinary and multiprofessional ways of working have been an important component of day-to-day activities. For many of the PHCTs, the workshop programme is the first opportunity to take time to plan together. Feedback still suggests that, for many PHCTs, practice meetings are a rare event. In other teams, whilst such meetings might take place, our experience suggests that they are not always very productive.

Evaluation of the PHCT programme

The programme was evaluated by Spratley, and the process has been described in detail elsewhere (Spratley, 1989). As the programme was multi-faceted, the evaluation had to take into account the many different dimensions involved. The information gathered by the evaluation programme was obtained from a variety of sources, both qualitative and quantitative. Spratley made a retrospective examination of the first five pilot PHCT workshops before the overall evaluation was introduced, including pre- and post-workshop questionnaires and practice visits undertaken by HEA workshop leaders. She attended planning meetings in order to observe the planning and organisation of the workshops, and she took part in a number of pre-workshop meetings designed to provide information about PHCT strategy.

Spratley also observed some PHCT workshops, in order to gain experience of the events, examine the functioning of the process, including the development of teamwork, and observe the production of plans and strategies. Information obtained as a result of locally organised evaluation activities, including questionnaires and feedback sheets, was analysed. Spratley participated in debriefing activities, primarily with the workshop planning teams, in order to reflect on the workshop events, PHCT progress and future developments, and to consider the outcome of local evaluations. Interviews were conducted with key individuals, including senior nurse managers, family practitioner committee (the forerunner of the family health service authority) administrators and other personnel, health education or promotion officers, HEA workshop leaders and primary care facilitators. These explored issues which emerged as a result of the evaluation, including the identification of both constraints and facilitating factors which might influence the development of PHCT plans.

Spratley attended various follow-up events for participating PHCTs some time after their workshop experience, in order to obtain feedback on their progress with their activities, including obstacles, challenges, successes and future plans. She also visited a number of PHCTs who had participated in the programme in order to learn at first hand something of their practice context and the way in which their plans had been developed, including any short-term outcomes. Finally, she took part in a number of LOT workshops in order to look at ways in which the PHCT workshop strategy might be taken forward on a self-sustaining basis in local areas. The evaluation was undertaken over a period of 1 year, and began with participation in the workshop organised in Trent Region in September 1988.

In summary, a number of research methods were used, including participant observation, interviews, documentary analysis and interactive approaches. Interim feedback, reflections and observations were fed back to planning groups so that they could use the information and experience which had been accumulating throughout the development of the MDTW programme as a whole, as well as reflecting on their own experience of organising such events.

Spratley found that the programme represented a robust and flexible framework for the development of health promotion initiatives in primary health care. The evaluation indicated that workshops provided a highly valued and much appreciated opportunity for those working in primary care to review and reflect on current activities, and to develop plans and strategies for disease prevention and health promotion initiatives. She suggested that the workshops enhanced communication, teamwork and practice organisation, and that they helped to clarify roles and responsibility in primary care. PHCTs not only enhanced their awareness of the potential which exists for the development of disease prevention and health promotion in PHC but, in addition, became more aware of the potential which exists for multidisciplinary and multiprofessional approaches to work. The plans that they developed, Spratley argued, reflected their determination to translate such insight into action on a day-to-day basis. She found that all those participating in the programme developed plans for disease prevention and health promotion. In some instances such plans updated ongoing activities, while in others they represented the creation of completely new initiatives. In yet other situations, these two approaches were combined. She indicated that the PHCTs greatly valued having the time and the opportunity to develop their plans as teams in a non-competitive setting. They also appreciated the emphasis that the workshops placed on the value of each member of the team, and the experience and expertise of each member. Plans developed by the PHCTs were felt by Spratley to demonstrate clearly an awareness of the need to assess, monitor and evaluate their activities. She suggested that, as a result of their involvement in the programme, the PHCTs were also able to identify opportunities for enhancing the involvement of the community in disease prevention and health promotion activities. In addition, Spratley looked at the LOTs.

In terms of planning, development, organisation and implementation of the programme, she felt that multiprofessional, multidisciplinary and multi-agency planning groups had been developed on a collaborative basis. This had enhanced local liaison between key planners and managers. Information and experience gained by a planning team in one context had, on some occasions, been taken up in another.

In addition, the content of the plans developed by the PHCTs was analysed and, wherever possible, linked to identified outcomes, either by an analysis of feedback gained at follow-up events or by visits made to practices. An important element of the methods used in the evaluation programme was the attempt to provide relevant and timely information at strategic points throughout the development of the programme, in order to describe and build upon the accumulating experience and maintain a dynamic aspect of the evaluation activities.

The main aim of the MDTW programme was to provide an opportunity for teams to develop their plans for disease prevention and health promotion, but health promotion is 'everybody's business', so an opportunity arose during the process to develop a sense of 'teamness'. Recent changes in primary care have led to larger PHCTs (see Chapter 3), and it is not unusual to have practices with 30, 40 or even 50 people. It is likely in this context that sub-groups are developed, e.g. a GP partners' team, a nursing team, or a team of professionals working together to address a specific health issue, such as asthma care. Although with such large numbers one cannot create a single team, I believe that one can develop in these organisations a shared philosophy of 'teamness', a shared way of working, a common practice objective or mission statement to which all members of the PHCT can subscribe.

The evaluation by Spratley (1989) demonstrated that, through the experience of working together on health promotion in the programme, PHCTs were able to develop in a number of areas. They were able to identify skills and resources which existed within the team, and to determine ways in which such skills could be used more effectively. In the workshops, participants appeared to take the opportunity to look at the strengths and weaknesses of their working situation and to devise strategies for meeting challenges and building on opportunities. A more equitable balance was also thought to be achieved in the team through the workshop process, which highlighted the equal value of each team member and his or her views.

Further research on the PHCT workshop programme was undertaken by Scott (1994). The study was conducted with the Ealing, Hammersmith and Hounslow LOTs, and focused on PHCT workshops held in 1993. The purpose of the study was to explore the nature of the relationships between community pharmacists and other PHCT members, and to assess the impact of community pharmacists' involvement in the PHCT workshop programme. The outcomes mirrored those of the earlier and much larger study. It was concluded that the involvement of community pharmacists in the PHCT workshop could have a beneficial effect on primary care integration and development, but that ultimately the degree of integration of the community pharmacists into the PHCT was limited by their reliance on pharmacy-based dispensing.

How successful is the programme?

The outcomes of this particular programme are many and varied. Some are easy to measure, e.g. whether a practice has produced an action plan or not. Some are more difficult to examine, e.g. how people feel about themselves in practice communication, administration and teamwork. My experience is mainly anecdotal and positive. The reader may well ask the following question: what about the negatives? Change and uncertainty can be painful for some people, whilst others thrive on it. The important factor to take into account is that it has been designed to facilitate team development in a safe environment where people are able to take risks. I believe that the successes or otherwise of this programme lie in the skills and knowledge of the workshop facilitators and the LOT, thorough preparation by the PHCTs prior to engaging in the programme, support during the programme, and the setting of realistic, achievable action plans.

As described earlier in this chapter, since the programmes began in 1987, primary care has experienced a number of changes. The support provided by the HEA National Unit for Health Promotion in Primary Care has attempted to reflect these changes and the resulting priorities. The MDTW Programme Team regularly receive feedback from visiting LOTs, telephone consultancy and advice, attendance at PHCT workshops, networking events and special events, e.g. opinion-seeking workshops and research projects. Two consensus workshops and a postal needs questionnaire have been instrumental in supporting the development of the programme. The process and outcomes of these exercises have been described in detail elsewhere (Health Education Authority, 1993, 1995a), but are summarised below.

Workshop 1 – February 1993

This event identified support and belief that the MDTW programme was an effective strategy for the development of PHCTs and their health promotion activities. LOT members expressed concern about the need to develop facilitation and group management skills. They recognised that they had knowledge and skills in primary care, but that these skills and knowledge were not sufficient to support team development. This preoccupation generated a need for training which LOTs felt should reflect the need of and be specific to the PHCTs. It was also suggested that a resource was needed to support the facilitation skills training – a facilitation skills 'toolbox'. It was suggested that the toolbox should contain materials which members of the LOT could dip into according to their experience and their needs. However, it was felt that the toolbox would be a framework which could then be built upon locally. Other types of toolbox were also suggested as necessary to support the PHCTs through current changes. LOT members said that they felt isolated, and they expressed a need for a newsletter and other opportunities to network and share experiences. In today's market-driven NHS culture, marketing skills and knowledge were also recognised as a priority.

These suggestions were taken forward by the National MDTW programme team. Representatives from 58 LOTs have since received training in group management, facilitation and techniques for teamworking in health promotion. These courses, supported by a group facilitation skills toolbox, are unique and have a content specific to primary health care and the LOT network. A newsletter for LOTs was developed in 1993, and a recent evaluation indicates that it is well received. The national MDTW programme team held a number of regional meetings (Health Education Authority, 1995b) to bring together colleagues involved in or of key influence to the programme for networking and debate. These meetings were intended to strengthen alliances nationally. A toolbox on managing change was developed for use by LOTs with PHCTs (Health Education Authority, 1995c). The training that accompanies the toolbox has to date been attended by representatives from 42 LOTs. A series of marketing workshops developed by the national team has been attended by representatives from 30 LOTs. All LOTs have been offered support for marketing the programme both to PHCTs and to key planners and managers.

Workshop 2 – June 1994

The participants in this workshop highlighted their continued support for the programme in providing a forum for developing health promotion and team-building for PHCTs. Marketing and increasing awareness among participants and key planners and managers, NHS Executive and Government were still a priority. The funding of the programme remained an issue for many LOTs. The facilitation and group management skills training and toolbox were valued, but the need for continued training to reflect the changing needs of LOTs was emphasised. Further research was needed on the advantages and disadvantages of the different models of team development, the benefits of teamworking, ways of measuring team effectiveness and the benefits of a team approach to health promotion in primary care. The national MDTW programme is currently engaged in addressing the above issues, and further information can be obtained from the MDTW.[6.1]

Conclusions

Disease prevention and health promotion activities are a central part of strategic thinking. The MDTW programme has been identified as an important mechanism for supporting such activities, particularly by Health Commissions. A positive outcome of this programme has been increased communication and liaison between the different members and agencies of the LOTs. The planning process for the programme depends to a large extent on the commitment of what in some cases may be quite a small number of individuals. Funding arrangements for the programme continue to cause difficulties for local organisers. Not all of those involved have been receptive to the principles on which the programme is based and their potential for the development of PHCTs. There has also been a lack of understanding in some cases with regard to the length of time required to create a sense of teamness and commitment to working together. The programme has changed in structure over time, with increased emphasis being placed on the importance of the pre- and post-workshop activities and the style of facilitation used to support team development.

The emergence of training and support for LOTs as part of the long-term development of the strategy is ongoing. As the membership of a LOT changes, training and support continue to be provided. In order to sustain a programme like this, it is important to take advantage of the potential which exists in contacts between LOT members and PHCTs, and to recruit new members widely.

For PHCT development, interventions must, as far as possible, be pragmatic and relevant to the experience of those working in primary health care, acknowledging the challenges and opportunities that exist. This has been demonstrated in feedback from PHCT workshops and in the two consensus workshops, and has been utilised in the form of the group management and facilitation skills training and toolbox. PHCTs with their busy work schedules appreciate having a structured task with an identified outcome – in this programme, the production of a plan to develop both their team and their health promotion and disease prevention activities.

Editors' summary

Gooding's chapter has outlined another of the key programmes in teambuilding in the late 1980s and the 1990s, giving a broad overview of the Health Education Authority's scheme and its evaluation. In many ways this chapter describes the way in which a fairly centralised model can adapt and develop in response to both policy change and local expediency. The evaluation indicates that the HEA programme was broadly successful in stimulating interdisciplinary working, particularly in the area of health promotion, suggesting that further work could utilise this approach.

Endnote

6.1. MDTW Programme Manager, HEA National Unit for Health Promotion in Primary Care, Block 10, The Churchill, Radcliffe Trust, Headington, Oxford OX3 7LJ, UK.

References

Acheson Report (1981) *London Health Planning Consortium: Primary Health Care in Inner London*. HMSO, London.

Department of Health (1989a) *General Practice in the National Health Service: The 1990 Contract*. Health Departments of Great Britain, London.

Department of Health (1989b) *Caring for People: Community Care in the Next Decade and Beyond*. Cm 849. HMSO, London.

Department of Health (1992) *The Patient's Charter*. HMSO, London.

Department of Health and Social Security (1981) *The Primary Health Care Team: A Report of a Joint Working Group of the Standing Medical Advisory Committee and the Standing Nursing and Midwifery Advisory Committee (The Harding Report)*. HMSO, London.

Department of Health and Social Security (1986) *Neighbourhood Nursing: A Focus For Care (Cumberlege Report)*. Department of Health and Social Security, London.

Health Education Authority (1993) *Multidisciplinary Team Workshop Programme: A Report on the Consensus Workshop Convened on 10 February 1993*. Health Education Authority, London.

Health Education Authority (1994) *Group Facilitation Skills Toolbox: Resources and Manual for Use with Primary Health Care Teams*. Health Education Authority, London.

Health Education Authority (1995a) *Multidisciplinary Team Workshop Programme: A Report on the Strategy and Development Workshop Convened on 17 June 1994*. Health Education Authority, London.

Health Education Authority (1995b) *Health Promotion in Primary Care – The Way Forward: Report on Two One-Day Networking Events for Purchasers and Providers of Health Promotion in Primary Care*. Health Education Authority, London.

Health Education Authority (1995c) *Managing Change Toolbox: A Resource for Local Organising Team Members to Use with Primary Health Care Teams*. Health Education Authority, London.

Kolb D (1984) *Experiential Learning*. Prentice Hall, Englewood Cliffs.

National Health Service Management Executive (1993) GP Contract Health Promotion Package: guidance on implementation to regional general managers and FHSA general managers. *NHS Letter* 93, 3.

Scott K (1994) *Involvement of Community Pharmacists in HEA Primary Health Care Team Workshops: A Pilot Study*. Health Education Authority, London, unpublished research.

Secretaries of State for Health, Wales, Northern Ireland and Scotland (1989) *Working for Patients*. HMSO, London.

Spratley J (1989) *Disease Prevention and Health Promotion in Primary Health Care: An Evaluation Report*. Health Education Authority, London.

7

The practice manifesto – a vehicle for promoting teamwork?

Debbie Freake and Tim van Zwanenberg

Introduction

A properly functioning team shares a common purpose (Gilmore *et al.*, 1974; Pritchard and Pritchard, 1992; Waine, 1992). Team members have a clear understanding of their own and other team members' roles and responsibilities, so the team can pool their knowledge, skills and resources (Gilmore *et al.*, 1974; Brown and van Zwanenberg, 1989; Waine, 1992). Their aims and objectives are explicit. However, it is not just the aims and objectives which are important – the process by which a team works together to complete and review them is equally critical.

The primary health care team (PHCT) at Adelaide Medical Centre, an inner city practice in Newcastle upon Tyne, sought to develop a sense of direction by drawing up a mission statement and a team manifesto (Adelaide Medical Centre Primary Health Care Team, 1991). The exercise started in 1989, well in advance of the government charter initiative. The perceived benefits have been validated by the experience of practices who have drawn up Primary Care Charters. This chapter examines the development of explicit aims and objectives with particular reference to the Adelaide Medical Centre. It reviews the development of their manifesto and achieved outcomes, setting these in the context of Primary Care Charters.

A primary health care manifesto – Adelaide Medical Centre primary health care team

> Come Friday I don't feel as though we've achieved anything.

This chance remark made by a receptionist in an inner city general practice was the start of 2 years of work for the PHCT in formulating a written declaration of intent with explicit objectives. Seven years later, the 'manifesto' remains at the heart of the practice. It has been revised several times, although it remains in essence little changed from the original version. The team decided that the constraints of a demand-led service meant that team members had little sense of direction and even less feeling of achievement. The practice manifesto arose from their desire to define the service that they wished to deliver. They believed that a manifesto drawn up by the primary health care team itself would help them to work towards common goals, and thought that the manifesto would focus their work, foster teamwork and provide a tool for evaluating success.

The process

It took 2 years of sporadic meetings for the task to be completed. Time was set aside on occasion during the weekly team meetings to work on the manifesto. (The PHCT meetings were, and still are, attended by as many team members as possible, including clinical and administrative staff, attached staff, students and trainees. They serve as a means of communication and education, and as a forum for discussion and decision-making, and they are regarded as an important part of the working week.) The production of the manifesto was time-consuming for all team members, but the meetings allowed members to air their ideas and views. Progress was intermittently hampered by such problems as a lack of direction, waning enthusiasm of the group, conflicting priorities, pressure on time, and staff changes. Lack of a feeling of 'ownership' of the manifesto among some team members, and the feeling that there was too great a concentration on detail, were also significant barriers. An absolute requirement was that the manifesto should be realistic, practical and achievable.

Most of the objectives were developed in meetings of the whole team, although those concerning prescribing were produced by the doctors alone. Consideration was given to mechanisms for audit of the various sections, and protocols were compiled where necessary. A careful record of the deliberations was kept, and from this one team member ultimately drew up a draft manifesto. After more detailed debate, the team felt confident that they could match the standards set in the manifesto.

The manifesto was included in the annual report, with copies distributed to team members, the local Family Health Services Authority (FHSA) and other interested parties. The manifesto was also displayed in folders in the practice waiting-area. Patients could ask for their own copy as advertised in the waiting-room, although few took up this offer. The manifesto soon proved to be useful induction material for trainees and new team members. It was used as a basis for individual appraisal, as well as providing a means whereby team members could understand the roles of others. It provided a framework for subsequent annual reports, and a systematic approach to audit was made explicit. The manifesto represented the beginnings of a strategic plan (see Appendix 7.1).

The manifesto revisited

In 1992, the manifesto was revised by a small working group consisting of two doctors and the practice nurse. Only the practice nurse had been a member of the practice when the original manifesto was compiled. Suggestions for change were taken back to the full team for discussion and agreement. The revision was important not only in returning ownership of the manifesto to the changed team, but also as a response to evolving community expectations and the changing nature of general practice. The main aims and objectives of the manifesto remained intact, the only significant change being a commitment to more active promotion of education and self-help, and a drive to improve relationships both within the team and with patients.

Three years later, in 1995, the team was surveyed about the manifesto by means of a self-completed questionnaire, and the results were used as a basis for further discussion. Of the 15 team members, three who had joined within the preceding 12 months were unaware of the manifesto. Two other members were aware of its existence, but had not read it before completing the questionnaire. Only four individuals had been members of the team throughout. When asked what the manifesto meant to individual team members, and to the team as a whole, the response was positive.

What team members said

> It is a sign that the practice cares and is committed to providing the best service possible.

> ... philosophy of the team ...

> ... culture of shared aims ...

> ... statement of intent ...

> ... improves cohesion and teamwork ...

> ... gives direction ...

> ... useful reference guide ...

> ... guidelines ...

> ... minimum achievable standards ...

> ... dissects the practice's activities and provides a framework for evaluation ...

Those members who were familiar with the manifesto felt that it influenced their day-to-day work, the work of the team as a whole, and the way in which the practice was perceived by the outside world. All team members considered that the aims and objectives of the revised manifesto remained relevant. Team members saw little connection between the manifesto and practice charters, and one of them dismissed the Patient's Charter as 'government rhetoric'.

Some additions and changes were suggested, including a greater commitment to a systematic audit programme, the development of a computerised chronic disease register, and the resurrection of regular staff appraisal. This most recent revision has, in particular, attempted to address one of the recognised limitations.

> In the current more aggressive business climate, primary care teams may need to consider the need for proactively seeking out patients' views, such as market research, focus groups and individual interviews.
> (Adelaide Medical Centre Primary Health Care Team, 1991)

A small working group involving a doctor, a practice nurse and a practice manager has been formed to address patient involvement and implement an in-house complaints system, the latter being a statutory requirement from April 1996. A Practice Charter outlining what patients can expect from the practice, and what the practice expects from its patients, has been sent to every patient.

To obtain maximum benefit, the manifesto must be monitored. Some objectives have been audited, either in response to a specific problem or as part of undergraduate or postgraduate teaching. For example, the repeat-prescribing system and medication reviews were identified as areas that caused frustration to the secretaries. Following the collection and analysis of prospective data by the trainee and secretary, the system was thoroughly overhauled. Monitoring of long-term medication (objective 2.8) can now be more easily and consistently achieved (see Appendix 7.1).

Some of the original manifesto objectives have been removed or amended. For example, biochemical thyroid function tests are no longer routinely used for annual monitoring of hypothyroid patients, and the manifesto has been altered accordingly.

Although the team has not systematically audited all of the objectives, the practice annual report addresses each of the areas covered and compares annual figures reflecting workload and health promotion. Risk factors for CHD, the care of diabetes and asthma, immunisations, cervical cytology, contraception, antenatal care, minor surgery, referrals to secondary care and deaths are all routinely audited each spring in preparation for the report.

The practice team at Adelaide Medical Centre believe that clear benefits have resulted from the production of the manifesto, and for them the process of discussion, writing and reviewing has been as important as the document itself (Table 7.1).

Table 7.1 Positive outcomes identified by the PHCT as a result of developing the 'manifesto'

Process	End result
• Improved team cohesion	• Sense of direction
• Improved understanding of differing ways of working	• Public declaration of intent
• Improved communication	• Reference guidelines
• Resolution of personal and professional conflict	• Clarification of roles and responsibilities
• Maintained commitment	• Framework for audit

Discussion

Teamworking and the need for common objectives

There has been considerable change since Professor John Brotherton's description of general practice as a 'cottage industry'. The traditional single-handed practitioner of 40 years ago, unsupported except by his wife, has now been replaced by a multidisciplinary primary health care team (Jarman and Cumberlege, 1987; Kuennsberg, 1991) (see also Chapter 3). However, there is more to a team than a collection of individuals working with the same client group or from the same building. The purpose of teamwork is to achieve a better outcome than that which would be achieved as the sum of individual and uncoordinated efforts.

The Harding Committee defined the primary health care team as:

> an independent group of medical practitioners, secretaries, health visitors, district nurses and midwives who share a common purpose and responsibility, each member clearly understanding his/her function and those of other members, so that all pool skills and knowledge to provide an effective primary health care service.
>
> (Department of Health and Social Security, 1981)

Yet lack of common objectives has long been identified as the main obstacle to the development of teamwork in primary health care (Marsh and Kaim-Caudle, 1976). Øvretveit (1993) also cites lack of common awareness of agreed priorities and ways of implementing priorities as one of a number of problems encountered in formal teams. He proposes five essentials for ensuring and improving co-operation in formal teams:

- manager or management group responsible for team performance;
- team accountability reviews;
- defined team leader position;
- team operational policy;
- team base.

Clarification of the overall aims of the team – or the team 'mission statement' – should be the first task. Some would argue that, by definition, a team has an operational policy, whether that is explicit or merely assumed. The advantages of an explicit policy are that it is readily available as guidance to all team members (especially those joining an established team), and that it ensures clear and agreed procedures, e.g. for patient management, staff appraisal and trainee teaching. It explains and publicises the purpose and organisation of the team, both to the general public and to management, and it provides a framework for evaluation of the team's performance (Øvretveit, 1993).

As long ago as 1986 the Cumberlege Report proposed that practices should have a written agreement with their attached community nurses (Department of Health and Social Security, 1986). A Department of Health task group established to consider the future of nursing services in the context of primary health care stated that: 'Teamwork with shared vision, shared objectives and, where appropriate, shared protocols, is essential if the range of skills and the resources to deploy them are to be channelled to the maximum benefit of people in the most cost-effective ways.'

From the study described in Chapter 12, which explored perceptions of successful team functioning, the following four indicators emerged as being particularly important:

- agreed aims and objectives;
- effective communication;
- patients receiving the best possible care;
- individual roles defined and understood.

The survey showed that there was agreement that aims and objectives should be set and recognised by all team members, adhered to, and regularly reviewed (Pearson and Spencer, 1995). In another study, 73 per cent of respondents agreed that the primary health care team should work to jointly agreed written objectives. There was also a high level of agreement among respondents about the aspects of care that should be provided as a minimum, with no significant differences between disciplines, suggesting that teams could be confident in identifying joint objectives (Pearson and van Zwanenberg, 1991).

However, other work has shown that in many teams members do not have explicit goals (Field and West, 1995). Furthermore, it appears that teams have resisted developing the kind of operational policies and service standards now common in industry, perhaps due to unease with the business-like approach to patients (Helme and Duerden, 1993). With the advent of the Patient's Charter, however, teams are increasingly making explicit their aims and objectives.

Although the Patient's Charter is viewed by some as a public relations exercise designed to distract attention from an unpopular government, those who have produced charters claim to have derived benefit from them. The principles underlying Practice Charters are based on teamwork theory, and are tied in to the production of a framework for practice development, such as the Adelaide Practice Manifesto. The charter approach can take the manifesto aims (of working towards common goals, achieving high standards and fostering teamwork) a step further by shifting the focus from within to without the team, and on to the patients themselves.

Primary Care Charters

A charter is a statement of principles, usually incorporating both rights and standards. It was originally the formal deed by which sovereigns guaranteed the rights and privileges of their subjects. The concept of health care charters was first introduced in the USA in the 1970s to support consumers' rights and their need for protection in the health care market. In the UK, the formation of the National Hospital Advisory Service in 1969, the Community Health Councils in 1974 and the Mental Health Act Commission in 1983 have all been symptomatic of the trend towards informing and protecting consumers. Voluntary organisations began to produce charters in the 1980s, e.g. the Charter for Children in Hospital in 1984. The Association of Community Health Councils in England and Wales produced their Patient's Charter in 1986.

Since then, many more charters have been produced by consumer groups, and all public services have published charters following the launch of the Citizen's Charter in 1990. The Patient's Charter was part of an overall strategy to improve the quality of services for patients. It incorporates the concepts of 'rights' and 'standards'. A *right* is defined by the Department of Health as 'a level of service to which the patient is entitled and which must always be delivered', whereas a *standard* is 'a level of service which the patient can expect to be delivered other than in exceptional circumstances' – in other words, 'standards' are aspirations which may not always be achieved.

The Patient's Charter describes ten rights and nine standards (Department of Health, 1991). In common with the national Charter, the local charters which followed were generally developed with minimal input from patients. Charters in primary care have not been compulsory, and have developed more slowly. The concept of informing patients of their responsibilities as well as their rights was introduced for the first time. Charters may reflect a change in the nature of the doctor–patient relationship from paternalistic to consumerist. The doctor–patient relationship is personal, continuing, and based on mutual trust. Some fear it may be jeopardised by notions of rights, standards and responsibilities.

Primary care charters aim to build a partnership between PHCTs and patients, based on an explicit understanding of the rights and responsibilities of each. A charter can help to define a practice's roles in the community. It can be seen as a sign of intent to provide the highest possible standards of service, and it is the logical external manifestation of a commitment to patient-centred care. The development of a charter requires consultation with patients and mechanisms for feedback. At their best, charters could improve the quality of services and give patients a voice.

Primary health care workers have recognised the need to include patients in individual management decisions but the involvement of patients in policy decisions has not been achieved easily. The manifesto developed by the PHCT at Adelaide Medical Centre was produced without consultation with patients, and feedback mechanisms produced little or no response. Increasingly, the team acknowledges that both are required, but appropriate mechanisms are still not in place. This may be partly explained by work pressures, but may also reflect nervousness about the process. Health professionals may fear unrealistic expectations and criticism from patients who are perceived to have a limited understanding of the issues. Such 'accountability' raises concerns about loss of professional autonomy.

However, patients' views can improve understanding between professionals, as well as enhancing the clinician–patient relationship. By focusing on the user–worker interface, and by measuring its effectiveness, work becomes 'task-centred' rather than tied by service boundaries. Barriers can be broken down by tackling shared problems. Users invariably add another dimension. Some argue that patients and their carers are a vital part of the health care team. Membership, of course, varies depending upon the task. Functionally the PHCT is 'a highly flexible organisation whose members form and dissolve multiple, overlapping and interlinking microteams' (Usherwood, 1993) in response to perceived needs. Patients fit more easily into this notion of 'microteams', which is also a useful concept for larger PHCTs where the development of aims and objectives inevitably falls to smaller more manageable groups.

The team at Adelaide Medical Centre is relatively small, serving a population of only 3700. Even in a team of this size, however, smaller microteams develop. For example, child protection issues are largely managed by one of the doctors and the two part-time health visitors. Diabetic care is mostly shared between another doctor and the practice nurse. In common with other PHCTs, microteams at Adelaide Medical Centre are responsible for development as well as for delivering most of the care. Consultation with users in such discrete areas may prove more practical and less daunting.

Conclusions

Manifestos and charters are about more than just the setting of aims and objectives. Reported benefits include greater team cohesiveness, motivation and morale, more effective communication, and clarification of different roles, assumptions and expectations (Hogg, 1994). Patient involvement provides an additional and advantageous perspective.

Editors' summary _____

Freake and van Zwanenberg have outlined their experiences with a very practical approach to integrating team goals through a practice manifesto, and have drawn some comparisons with the national move towards patient charters. They have demonstrated a number of benefits for team members. Most importantly, they have argued that patients should have a clear voice in policy decisions, so that the patients themselves become contributing members of the team.

Appendix 7.1 – Adelaide Medical Centre Manifesto

(revised Spring 1995)

Aims

1.1   To provide an accessible high standard of primary health care that adapts to the needs of our patients.
1.2   To work together and support each other as a team.
1.3   To educate ourselves, our colleagues, trainees and students from any discipline.
1.4   To promote and facilitate our patients' own health care through advice, education and counselling and, where necessary, to act as their advocate.
1.5   To maintain close links with the community within which we work.

Objectives

The following objectives were stated.

Acute care

1.1   On weekdays, patients with non-urgent problems will be seen at the surgery (as agreed with the patient) within 24 hours of their request.
1.2   Patients with non-urgent problems will be offered an appointment with the doctor of their choice within 1 week of their request (except when that doctor is away).
1.3   At any time, patients with urgent problems (as perceived by the patient) will be advised by a doctor as soon as is practical, and seen as necessary, either at home or in the surgery (as agreed with the patient).
1.4   Through the receptionist, patients will be able to contact the practice nurse, district nurse, health visitor, community midwife and dietitian.
1.5   Advice will be available by telephone, and patients will be encouraged to use self-help where appropriate.

Prescribing

2.1   As a general rule, all drugs except combination preparations will be prescribed generically by doctors using their own prescription pads.

2.2   The doctors will strive to comply with *A Basic Formulary for General Practice*, and will regularly review their prescribing with the aid of Prescribing Analysis and Costs (PACT).

2.3   Trainees will prescribe on partner A's prescription pad using the 'D' facility.

2.4   Potential and known drug abusers will not, where possible, be given prescriptions for drugs that can be abused.

2.5   Benzodiazepines will not be prescribed *de novo* except in exceptional circumstances, and long-term users will be encouraged to withdraw from the drug.

2.6   Appetite suppressants will not be prescribed.

2.7   Unnecessary prescribing (e.g. antibiotics to treat viral illness) will be avoided, patients will be encouraged to use simple, symptomatic treatments for common self-limiting conditions, and alternative coping strategies will be explored.

2.8   Patients on long-term medication will be monitored closely and reviewed at appropriate intervals.

Women's health

3.1   Women will be offered the full range of contraceptive services, provided by a woman doctor if desired.

3.2   Pregnant women will be offered shared antenatal and postnatal care.

3.3   Requests for home confinement will be considered individually.

3.4   Women aged 20–70 years will be offered a cervical smear test every 3 years (unless inappropriate) until they have had two normal post-menopausal smears and are aged 65 years, as dictated by current DoH guidelines.

3.5   Education and advice concerning the menopause will be available for all women, and hormone replacement therapy will be considered for individual women.

3.6   Breast awareness information will be available to and such awareness will be encouraged in all women. Participation in the breast screening programme will also be actively encouraged.

Health promotion and preventative care

4.1   All children (whose parents have given consent) will be fully immunised, and screened at the appropriate intervals for treatable undetected conditions.

4.2   The weekly baby clinic, run by a health visitor and a doctor, will address all child health issues, including developmental and safety aspects, and will provide a setting in which any other concerns can be raised.

4.3   All adults aged over 16 years will be screened opportunistically for coronary heart disease risk factors as appropriate, prioritising those most at risk, and will be offered appropriate advice on lifestyle changes.

4.4   All patients over 75 years of age will be functionally assessed annually.

4.5   Patients intending to travel abroad will be given appropriate advice and immunisation, and identified problems dealt with appropriately.

4.6   We shall be proactive in our approach to our patients' sexual health, including our young patients.

Chronic care

5.1   We shall endeavour to offer each diabetic, asthmatic and hypertensive patient a programme of structured care in the surgery or at home according to practice protocols, in collaboration with colleagues.

5.2   All patients with ongoing physical and mental health problems will be regularly reviewed at appropriate intervals.

Terminal care

6.1   Patients with terminal illnesses, and their families, will be fully supported in the community by the practice team.

6.2   Bereaved relatives will be visited soon after the patient's death.

Patient relations

7.1   Any patient living within the practice boundaries and wishing to register will meet a doctor and be provided with a practice information leaflet.

7.2   Maintenance of continuity of patient care will be considered a major priority.

7.3   The team will endeavour to maintain contact with or visit hospitalised patients.

7.4   Health education will be encouraged by the use of poster displays, information leaflets and practice library books.

7.5   Patients will be able to see information held about themselves on the computer, on request. Written records from November 1991 onward will also be made available.

7.6   Suggestions from patients will be welcomed. Complaints will be discussed openly, taken seriously, and responded to promptly according to the practice complaints procedure. Periodic surveys of patient views will be carried out.

7.7   The staff will endeavour to ensure that patients are treated courteously and sympathetically at all times, and in return the staff will expect to be treated in a similar manner by the patients.

7.8   The staff will endeavour to ensure that waiting time is kept to a minimum.

Teamwork

8.1 Each team member will be offered feedback and discussion as a means of personal development at least once yearly.
8.2 Each team member will be encouraged to pursue his or her own further education and training and to take part in in-house training and team training.
8.3 All team members will be able to communicate freely and be respected as an integral part of the whole.
8.4 There will be regular meetings, *ad hoc* meetings for sub-groups, away-days and occasional social outings.

Teaching

9.1 The trainee will have at least one and preferably two protected teaching sessions with a principal each week.
9.2 A principal will be available at all times to provide support and guidance for the trainee.
9.3 The team will endeavour to ensure that University commitments do not encroach upon the standard of care provided for our patients (whilst supporting those with multiple commitments).
9.4 Patients will be given an informed choice with regard to involvement in research and teaching.

Audit and information

10.1 All records will be summarised, and screening cards regularly updated.
10.2 Manual registers will be maintained for births, deaths, malignant disease, minor surgical operations and dangerous drugs. Computer registers will be maintained for births and specific diseases/problems.
10.3 Coronary heart disease risk factors, specific chronic diseases, diabetes and asthma care and geriatric review will be computerised and amenable to audit.
10.4 Trainees and medical students attached to the practice will be encouraged to undertake audit exercises as projects.
10.5 A regular, systematic audit system will be set up and maintained.
10.6 By June of each year an annual report will be produced, which will include a review of the objectives for consideration by the team.

NB This Appendix is reproduced with permission from the *British Journal of General Practice*.

References

Adelaide Medical Centre Primary Health Care Team (1991) A primary health care team manifesto. *British Journal of General Practice* 41, 31–3.

Brown C and van Zwanenberg TD (1989) Primary and community health services in Newcastle upon Tyne – a joint statement of intent. *Journal of the Royal College of General Practitioners* 39, 164–5.

Department of Health (1991) *The Patient's Charter*. Department of Health, London.

Department of Health and Social Security (1981) *The Harding Committee*. Department of Health and Social Security, London.

Department of Health and Social Security (1986) *Community Nursing Review: Neighbourhood Nursing: a Focus for Care*. The Cumberlege Report. Department of Health and Social Security, London.

Field R and West M (1995) Teamwork in primary health care. 2. Perspectives from practices. *Journal of Interprofessional Care* 9, 123–30.

Gilmore N, Bruce N and Hunt M (1974) *The Work of the Nursing Team in General Practice*. Council for Education and Training of Health Visitors, London.

Helme K and Duerden M (1993) Working towards 'Investor in People' for the Whickham practice: a case study. In Chan JFL (ed.) *Quality and Its Applications*, pp. 399–402. Penshaw, Sunderland.

Hogg C (1994) *Beyond the Patient's Charter: Working with Users*. Health Rights Ltd.

Jarman J and Cumberlege J (1987) Developing primary health care. *British Medical Journal* 294, 1005–8.

Kuennsberg EV (1991) The team in primary care (1983–1990) In *The Royal College of General Practitioners Members' Reference Book*, pp. 433–8. Sabrecrown Publishers, London.

Marsh GN and Kaim-Caudle P (1976) *Teamcare in General Practice*. Croom Helm, London.

Øvretveit J (1993) *Co-ordinating Community Care – Multidisciplinary Teams and Care Management*. Open University Press, Milton Keynes.

Pearson P and van Zwanenberg T (1991) *Who is the Primary Health Care Team? What Should They be Doing?* Department of Primary Health Care, University of Newcastle upon Tyne, Newcastle upon Tyne.

Pearson P and Spencer J (1995) Pointers to effective teamwork: exploring primary care. *Journal of Interprofessional Care* 9, 131–8.

Pritchard P and Pritchard J (1992) *Developing Teamwork in Primary Care*. Oxford University Press, Oxford.

Usherwood T (1993) The primary care organisation: team or hologram? *Journal of Interprofessional Care* 7, 211–16.

Waine C (1992) The primary care team. *British Journal of General Practice* 42, 498–9.

8

Achieving focused teamwork

John Spencer and Alice Southern

Introduction

In this chapter we describe a project which aimed to achieve focused teamwork in primary care through the medium of audit. In 1992, the Department of Health invited bids for funding of projects to examine the problems of multidisciplinary audit in primary care, and to produce a range of practical examples for wider dissemination. Several key areas were flagged for exploration, including resource needs, process and outcome measures, information requirements, record systems, and so on. The North Tyneside Multidisciplinary Audit Project was one of five successful bids (see also Chapter 9), and was a collaboration between five general practices, the North Tyneside Medical Audit Advisory Group (MAAG) and the Department of Primary Health Care at the University of Newcastle upon Tyne.

The project was based on the concept of a practice audit plan (Baker and Presley, 1990), using the framework of a practice manifesto (Adelaide Medical Centre Primary Health Care Team, 1991) (see also Chapter 7), and had the following aim:

> To support a number of North Tyneside primary health care teams in the development of practice audit plans, and to record and evaluate this process, thereby allowing dissemination to other North Tyneside teams and further afield.
>
> (Spencer *et al.*, 1993, p. 3)

The project 'philosophy' had two strands.

- It took a broad view of audit, as a process examining any aspect of practice, clinical or organisational, with a view to identifying opportunities for improvement.
- There was a fundamental emphasis on ensuring effective team functioning as a precursor to multidisciplinary audit.

A problem-orientated approach was adopted, and the method used to facilitate 'effective team function' was the practice 'away-day'.

Profile of North Tyneside

North Tyneside is a small, geographically discrete area at the mouth of the River Tyne, neighbouring the city of Newcastle upon Tyne to the west and South East Northumberland to the north. It is approximately 82 square kilometres in area, and has a population of about 195 000 inhabitants. At the time of the project, the district was served by 107 general practitioners in 35 practices (of which seven were single-handed) administered by North Tyneside Family Health Services Authority, and two district general hospitals. In the past, it had the reputation of having the highest prescribing costs in the UK in terms of average costs per patient. The district contains several pockets of socio-economic deprivation, including the Meadowell Estate (the scene of riots in 1991), as well as areas of affluence, such as Tynemouth.

Project protocol

Although the interventions were the same for all participating teams, a fundamental principle of the project was to work with the primary care teams' own agendas and priorities, and an action research approach was adopted in preference to an experimental model. The protocol for the project was as follows:

- recruitment of practices;
- baseline evaluation questionnaire administered to all team members;
- the first practice 'away-day';
- two practice visits by the project team;
- a support meeting for members of all participating teams;
- the second practice 'away-day';
- follow-up evaluation questionnaire administered to all team members.

It was hoped that, by the end of the project, each team would have produced a practice audit plan and would be in the process of implementing it. The project team consisted of an academic general practitioner, a nurse researcher with a health visiting background, a health psychologist and the MAAG facilitator.

The time scale for the project was tight (bids for funding were invited in August 1992; the project started in October 1992; the project ended on 31 March 1993; the report was submitted to the Department of Health in May 1993), which somewhat limited its scope. Every practice in the district (35 practices in total) was contacted and invited to participate. Seven practices responded and were visited by the project manager, who explained the project in more detail. Five practices finally agreed to take part, and their profiles are shown in Table 8.1.

Three of the practices had GP members on the MAAG, and all were active locally in medical politics, service development or education. None the less, only one practice had ever met as an entire team, although all of the practices held smaller meetings of one kind or another. The general practitioners, and in two practices the practice manager, were the team members with whom participation was negotiated.

Interventions

Four different interventions were employed.

'Away-days'

Two such sessions, lasting for around 5 hours each, were provided away from the practice, with an interval of approximately 4 months between them. The whole team was invited to attend, and both sessions were facilitated by the same person (the health psychologist, who had considerable experience of working with primary health care teams). Although structured to provide a forum for discussion in which all members could contribute equally, the content of the session reflected specific issues and observations raised by individuals.

On the first 'away-day', participants were encouraged to use the protected time to review the whole practice, including the service that it offered from both the professional and consumer perspective, the way in which it functioned in areas such as communication and decision-making, and the working environment it created for team members. A set of priorities that the team collectively felt should be improved was then agreed upon, and appropriate aims or standards were discussed. This was achieved by asking members to answer a series of open-ended questions about the practice which, through discussion in small groups, produced a set of observations. These were grouped under the following headings for feedback to the entire group: what encourages job satisfaction; tasks to do, things to change; general observations; things to be proud of. When considering 'tasks to do', a check-list of headings based on the practice manifesto (Adelaide Medical Centre Primary Health Team, 1991) was provided both to encourage a comprehensive review of 'where we are now', and as a template for a practice audit plan (Table 8.2; see also Chapter 7).

A similar format was used for the second 'away-day', with team members being encouraged to review progress and, again, to clarify what issues should be subjected to audit in the practice. Participants were also asked to reflect upon aspects of multidisciplinary audit in response to the following three questions. 'From your point of view, what makes the practice run well,

Table 8.1 Profiles of participating practices

Practice	List size	General practitioners	Practice manager	Receptionists	Secretaries	Computer operators	Practice nurses	Attached staff	Teaching/ training
A	5800	3 FT 1 PT 1 VT	1	3 PT	1 FT 1 PT	2	—	1 RGN 1 SEN 1 HV	1 MW	Training
B	8800	4 FT 2 PT	1	9 PT	—	—	1 FT 1 PT	1 RGN 1 SEN 2 HV	1 MW	Teaching
C	3650	2 FT	1	1 FT 4 PT	1 PT	—	2 PT	1 RGN 1 HV	1 MW 1 CPN 1 SW	Teaching
D	2700	1 FT	—	2 PT	1 FT	—	1 FT	1 RGN 1 HV	1 MW 2 Diet	—
E	2500	2 PT	—	1 FT 2 PT	—	—	1 PT	1 RGN 1 HV	1 MW	—

FT, full-time; PT, part-time; VT, vocational trainee; PM, practice manager; PN, practice nurse; RGN, registered general nurse; SW, social worker; Diet, dietitian; SEN, state enrolled nurse; HV, health visitor; MW, midwife; CPN, community psychiatric nurse.

All practices were computerized. Only one practice had met as a whole team, although all practices did have meetings of one type or another.

Table 8.2 Check-list for producing a practice audit plan

- Access
- Acute care
- Chronic disease management
- Screening
- Immunisation
- Drug use
- Information systems
- Female health
- Terminal care
- Business plan
- Patient relations

Derived from Adelaide Medical Centre Practice Manifesto
(Adelaide Primary Health Care Team, 1991).

and why?' 'What are the barriers or problems that tend to get in the way of
the practice improving its standards?' 'What are your thoughts about multidisciplinary audit, its advantages and disadvantages?' Each participant
answered these questions in his or her own words on paper, and these
responses were collected by the project team, analysed thematically and
collated.

About 2 weeks after the 'away-day' the lists were sent back to individual
team members, and each of the themes was rated on a Likert scale. Themes
were then ranked according to the summary score, the final ranking giving
an impression of what the team (as a group of individuals) regarded as
important issues in effective functioning, and how multidisciplinary audit
could aid this process. In a second, open-ended task, participants in groups
of eight or less were given about 20 minutes to produce a list of comments –
both positive and negative – about the entire project.

Practice visits

Four of the practices were visited on two occasions, and the fifth was visited
only once, by project team members over a period of 3 months. The aims of
these visits were firstly to provide an opportunity for practice team members
to reflect on the project in general, and on their own progress in particular,
and secondly to offer support and guidance if necessary. The visits lasted for
approximately 1 hour, they took place at lunchtime on practice premises, and
as many team members as were able to attend were invited. Notes were
taken by the project team.

Evening meeting

An evening meeting was held in the local Postgraduate Medical Centre. This
was facilitated by the project team, and provided an opportunity for

participating team members to report on progress and to share ideas and concerns about the project, or indeed about any aspect of teamwork, multi-disciplinary audit, etc., as appropriate. It took place approximately 2 months after the first 'away-day', in the middle of the second round of practice visits, and about 4 to 6 weeks before the second 'away-day'.

Continuing support

Continuing support was provided by one of the authors (Alice Southern) in her capacity as MAAG facilitator.

Evaluation

The aim of the evaluation was to describe the interventions, and to compare and contrast the activity of participating teams before and after the programme. It was based on the following sources of information:

- questionnaire surveys before and after the project (a self-completion questionnaire about team function and attitudes to audit; see below);
- a list of topics, problems and issues identified at the first 'away-day';
- progress reports from the teams (during practice visits, at the evening meeting and at the second 'away-day');
- responses to three questions about multidisciplinary audit at the second 'away-day';
- feedback about the project;
- observations of the project team.

Questionnaire survey

Prior to the first 'away-day' and about 2 weeks after the second one, a postal self-completion questionnaire was sent to all members of the participating teams. The initial baseline questionnaire was developed from an interview schedule used in previous evaluations of teambuilding interventions (Pearson, 1992; see also Chapter 10), and was divided into three sections covering the following areas:

- information about the practice, in particular the respondent's perceptions of how 'their' team functioned, using both open-ended questions and a group of questions (the 'Teamwork Scale') employing a 5-point attitudinal scale derived from previous work (Dyer, 1987) (the areas addressed are shown in Table 8.3);
- individuals' perceptions about audit, including their attitudes towards audit, whether they were already or would like to be involved in multi-disciplinary audit, and what problems they might encounter;
- what expectations respondents had of the 'away-days', what changes

Table 8.3 'Teamwork Scale' items included in the questionnaire

A	To what extent do I feel a real part of the team?
B	How safe is it in this team to be at ease, relaxed and myself?
C	To what extent do I feel 'under cover', that is, have private thoughts, unspoken reservations or unexpressed feelings and opinions that I have not felt comfortable bringing out into the open?
D	How effective are we, in our team, in getting out and using the ideas, opinions and information of all team members in making decisions?
E	To what extent are the goals the team is working towards understood, and to what extent do they have meaning for me?
F	How well does the team work at its tasks?
G	Our planning and the way in which we operate as a team are largely influenced by . . .
H	What is the level of responsibility for work in our team?
I	How are differences and conflicts handled in our team?
X	Where do we feel our team is at present (in terms of health care delivery)?

After Dyer, 1987.

they would like to see arising from them, and what concerns they had in anticipation of them.

The second questionnaire sent after the second 'away-day' reviewed the same areas and, in addition, asked what audit activity respondents had participated in and their reasons for non-involvement, as well as requesting feedback about the project interventions. Analysis was performed using the SPSS-PC software package (Norusis, 1988). In addition, thematic analysis of the open-ended questions and observational data were used.

Results

These have been published in full in the project report (Spencer *et al.*, 1993), and only selected data will be presented and discussed here, mostly as it relates to the issue of teamwork.

Questionnaire data

The responses to the two questionnaires by both individual teams and professional groups are shown in Figures 8.1 and 8.2.

In total, 88 per cent of respondents to the first questionnaire felt that they were part of a team. However, included among those who said no or were unsure were respondents whose job would generally be seen as central and integral to a PHCT's functioning, e.g. receptionists.

The 10 attitudinal questions were rated on a 5-point scale, the mean overall scores were calculated for each item, and the difference between each set of

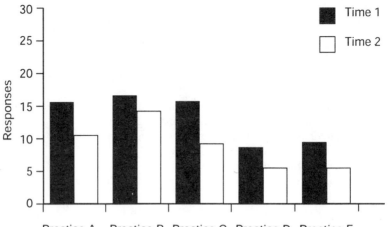

Figure 8.1

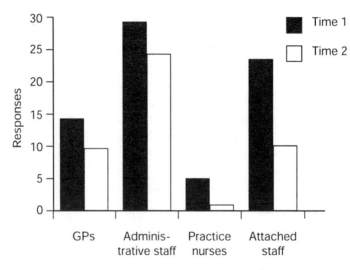

Figure 8.2

scores in the two questionnaires was tested for significance using *t*-tests. The statistically significant changes were an overall increase in 'understanding the team's goals' ($P < 0.05$) and in perceptions of 'influence in planning' ($P < 0.05$). For employed staff only (i.e. reception and administrative staff, and practice nurses) there was a significant decrease in the feeling of 'being able to be oneself' ($P < 0.05$), and for GPs there was a significant decrease in 'perceived level of responsibility for work' ($P < 0.01$).

In both questionnaires respondents were asked to describe specific occasions when they felt that their team had either been working well or not.

There were considerably more positive than negative responses in both questionnaires, reflecting favourably on the respondents' overall perceptions of team functioning in relation to the project. Some verbatim examples follow.

Project activities were often mentioned as situations where teams were felt to be working well, for example at the 'away-days', with 'time to draw up policy decisions on certain aspects of patients' care, such as policy for visiting patients discharged from hospital' or 'honest sharing of views in a safe, supportive environment'. Several examples of audit in practice apparently occurring as a consequence of the project were cited as positive aspects of teamwork. For example: 'for 2 weeks we all did an appointments audit for both practice nurse and doctor'.

Negative comments were mainly concerned with two issues:

- failures and problems due to limited resources, particularly associated with premises, e.g. 'the conditions in the health centre cause some problems';
- problems of communication, including both general communication, e.g. 'there has been a problem between receptionists in the morning and the afternoon, involving resentment of the amount of work done. Poor communication involved', and more specifically communication between doctors and other staff, e.g. '... the doctors made this task harder – there was no appreciation ...'.

Analysis of the membership of each team as perceived by individual respondents showed that doctors were viewed by all respondents as part of the primary health care team, whilst many other professionals, such as secretaries, were only occasionally mentioned. This parallels the findings of Pearson's study in Newcastle (see Chapter 10).

Understanding of the concept of audit before the project appeared to vary widely. Responses to the question 'I think audit is ...' ranged from a 'textbook' definition, such as 'assessing practice; setting standards; implementing change; monitoring standards', through quite sophisticated definitions that incorporated the concept of a cyclical review of practice with the aim of improving care, to expressions of ignorance – 'an unknown quantity to me' – or perceptions of audit as an external process – 'a check by a non-member of the team on how the team is performing, measured against the team's targets'. On the other hand, the majority of respondents said that they would be willing to take part in multidisciplinary audit. However, only 61 per cent of respondents to the second questionnaire felt that they had been involved in multidisciplinary audit during the course of the project. Problems experienced in undertaking multidisciplinary audit included several issues directly related to teamworking, e.g. poor communication within the team, and difficulties in implementing change and 'seeing things through'. None the less, multidisciplinary audit was considered by most respondents to foster a positive team spirit and enthusiasm, stimulating the team to take a broad view of its function, and involving everyone in the team in working towards common goals.

Topics and problems identified at the first 'away-day'

Unsurprisingly, these were diverse, and ranged from organisational and structural issues (e.g. appointment systems and waiting-room facilities) to aspects of clinical care (e.g. the need for protocols or 'asthma care'). They were generally focused on areas where work was felt to be needed to improve, directly or indirectly, either the quality of service for patients or the quality of the working environment for team members. Communication within the team, information handling and appointment systems emerged as major themes across all five practices.

Progress reports

Discussions with representatives of the participating teams during the two practice visits between 'away-days', and at the evening meeting, indicated that, on the whole, they were all progressing successfully with the development of audit in a variety of areas (e.g. appointment systems, repeat prescribing, follow-up of patients after discharge from hospital). In two practices, an 'audit care team' or 'practice audit group' had been set up, and a formal audit plan was being drawn up in at least three of the practices.

Feedback about the project

On the second 'away-day', participants were invited to give feedback about any aspect of the project. This was done in small groups, and then shared with the whole team. Verbatim comments were recorded, and the ratio of positive to negative comments was approximately 5:1. Comments about the project as a whole included the following: 'enabled us to look at ourselves in relation to other practices', 'useful ideas came out of it. More of a team approach' and, interestingly, 'felt in retrospect that the project had concentrated on teambuilding, not audit'.

With regard to the 'away-days', there were generally very positive comments about the benefits, including appreciation of other people's roles, the opportunity to 'plan as a team', and to involve everybody ('attached staff felt more involved and wanted to be more involved at other times'), and the prospect of the second 'away-day' 'made us try to conclude things'. There was also a widespread feeling that participants 'came away with lots of positive things about working together'.

Outcomes of the project

Three of the five teams produced a formal practice audit plan, although in only one case was this as detailed as proposed in the original protocol. A fourth practice drew up a practice manifesto which, it was proposed, would form the basis of an audit plan in the future. In two of the practices an audit group (multidisciplinary in nature) was established to spearhead the plans. By the end of the project, *all* of the teams had undertaken audit and review, resulting in change in at least some of the areas that they had identified for action. These included appointment systems, information handling (including information for patients), internal communication, repeat prescribing and specific clinical areas, e.g. hormone replacement therapy. Despite some problems and barriers, the advantages of multidisciplinary audit were perceived to include fostering team spirit and enthusiasm, stimulating the team to take an holistic view of the practice, involving everyone in the process, seeing things from other people's perspectives, and collaborative working to achieve common goals.

Discussion

Despite the problems with which primary health care teams are beset in terms of functioning effectively, it seemed self-evident that a group of professionals working together would periodically perceive the need to review their activities. In groups where objectives, goals or targets are defined, this would involve a review of progress towards their achievement. We used this broad notion of review of team functioning as the basis for this project. It is in fact closer to the concept of 'continuous quality improvement' (Berwick *et al.*, 1990) than the narrower idea of clinical audit.

A fundamental concept in quality management is that the main sources of defects lie in problems in the process, rather than with individuals. However, in solving problems, 'total employee involvement' is considered to be critical (Berwick *et al.*, 1990). Such involvement requires a working environment in which individuals feel confident and safe to be critical (or to be criticised), in which there is a sense of 'ownership', and in which individuals have as much understanding of the process(es) as possible. For this reason, we felt that effective team functioning was an essential prerequisite for successful multidisciplinary audit. In other words, we felt that we should approach the project from the starting point of team development rather than audit *per se*. Recent research has suggested that one of the most important factors influencing the participation of a primary health care team in multidisciplinary audit is the level of discussion within the practice, which is a major attribute of an effective team (Baker *et al.*, 1995a; see also Chapter 9).

Thus, whereas the main aim of the project was to facilitate the production of comprehensive audit plans by the practices, we realised from the start that, given the time scale of the project (6 months, including the Christmas holiday), much of the work would be simply facilitating team function. The methods used ('away-days', practice visits and meetings) were explicitly focused on the teams' own agendas, with the aim of helping them to achieve a broad perspective and to identify important issues for review in the practice. In this way we felt that any subsequent review, or audit, would be more likely to be 'worker-centred, practice-based and problem-orientated' (Baker and Presley, 1990). In the language of 'continuous quality improvement', we hoped that the method would provide an opportunity for participants to gain a greater understanding of 'processes' at the same time as promoting a climate of ownership, participative safety, and so on, through a form of 'total employee involvement' (Berwick *et al.*, 1990). The project was only partially successful, in that only three of the five participating practices produced practice audit plans, although a fourth practice drew up a set of objectives in the form of a manifesto, and *all* of the practices undertook audit projects of a multidisciplinary nature.

However, in terms of facilitating team function and helping to create a climate in which multidisciplinary audit is more likely to occur, we felt that we had been successful. Responses to the teamwork scale questions showed changes in all practices in terms of understanding team goals and of perceived influence on planning, both of which are key factors in change management (Spiegal *et al.*, 1992). Obviously we were only observing changes in individuals' perceptions of team functioning, rather than objective changes in team effectiveness.

Team effectiveness can be conceptualised as the capacity of a team to survive, adapt, maintain itself and grow (see Chapter 11). 'Team innovativeness' has been proposed as an important dimension of team effectiveness, an innovation in this context being 'the introduction and application of new and improved ways of working in a team setting' (Poulton and West, 1993) – a definition that would embrace the concept of multidisciplinary audit. Four criteria are important if a team is to be innovative: shared objectives; 'participative safety' (i.e. a supportive, co-operative and non-threatening climate); a commitment to excellence; and support within the team for innovation and change. Predictors of team innovativeness include high levels of collaboration within the team, a commitment to common objectives, and a climate for innovation.

Perhaps more than anything else, audit (and quality) is about innovation and change, especially in the multidisciplinary setting. The relationship between effective team functioning and successful multidisciplinary audit is in many respects one of 'chicken and egg'. However, in this project we took team functioning as the starting point because we were concerned that audit may not be the best place to start when a team is not developed, since it may prove a risky venture with a high probability of failure (Humphrey and Hughes, 1992). In the words of Firth-Cozens 'If audit – clinical or medical – is to progress . . . we need to learn how to create teams and how to work within them' (Firth-Cozens, 1992). As she observes, multidisciplinary audit involves 'an exploration of uncharted ground' which will require new skills in each team member. More recently, the report of the Primary Care Clinical Audit

Working Group of the Chief Medical Officer's Clinical Outcomes Group echoed these sentiments thus: 'Making multidisciplinary practice teams work effectively, and managing change constructively, will invariably be more testing than mastering the technicalities of the audit process' (Primary Care Clinical Audit Working Group of Clinical Outcomes Group, 1994).

There is evidence that teambuilding interventions such as 'away-days' will be most effective if they are focused on specific areas (such as problem-solving), and that it is unrealistic to expect change in anything other than small increments (West, 1993). It is also becoming clear that most primary health care teams will require support and facilitation to undertake comprehensive multidisciplinary audit (Baker *et al.*, 1995b), although some teams may be functioning sufficiently well to be able to 'go it alone' (Lawrence, 1992).

Conclusions

Since the end of the project, the programme of team 'away-days' focused on quality issues has continued and developed. Almost two-thirds of North Tyneside practices have attended one or more 'away-days', and in a recent evaluation of North Tyneside MAAG activities which examined the views of PHCT members, the majority of respondents had found the away-days useful and stimulating. Comments such as 'reflective thinking, initiated audit' and 'changed my practice and improved rapport within the PHCT' give a flavour of the largely positive responses (McElroy *et al.*, 1996).

The project thus achieved its aims, the main output being a simple model for facilitating teamwork as a prelude to undertaking multidisciplinary audit. The method we used seemed to promote 'team innovativeness' and to help to create a climate in which multidisciplinary audit was more likely to be undertaken. One of the dangers of development work of this kind is that it is assumed that only exceptional teams act as a testbed, and that pilot schemes are not transferable. The continuation of this approach since the initial pilot demonstrates that it *is* transferable, and that it is valued by a wide range of practices. Further research is needed to explore the impact of multidisciplinary audit on patient care.

Editors' summary

In this chapter, Spencer and Southern have considered an initiative which was designed to develop multidisciplinary approaches to quality improvement in primary health care. They have drawn attention to the need to focus on involving team members from the beginning in any attempt to change practice. The intervention described was found to be successful in stimulating audit and review of practice in five teams within a single district. The project also demonstrates the potential of sharing ideas and findings between practices in a locality.

References

Adelaide Medical Centre Primary Health Care Team (1991) A primary health care team manifesto. *British Journal of General Practice* 41, 31–3.

Baker R and Presley P (1990) *The Practice Audit Plan.* Royal College of General Practitioners, Bristol.

Baker R, Robertson N and Farooqi A (1995a) Audit in general practice: factors influencing participation. *British Medical Journal* 311, 31–4.

Baker R, Sorrie R, Reddish S, Hearnshaw H and Robertson N (1995b) The facilitation of clinical audit in primary health care teams – from audit to quality assurance. *Journal of Interprofessional Care* 9, 237–44.

Berwick DM, Godfrey AB and Roessner J (1990) *Curing Health Care. New Strategies for Quality Improvement.* Jossey-Bass, San Francisco.

Dyer W (1987) *Teambuilding: Issues and Alternatives.* Addison-Wesley, Reading, MA.

Firth-Cozens J (1992) Building teams for effective audit. *Quality in Health Care* 1, 252–5.

Humphrey C and Hughes J (1992) *Audit and Development in Primary Care.* Kings' Fund, London.

Lawrence M (1992) Audit and TQM in diabetic care in general practice. *Quality in Health Care* 1 (Supplement), S20–21.

McElroy H, Spencer J and Thomson R (1996) *Evaluation of the North Tyneside Medical Audit Advisory Group – Views of Primary Health Care Teams, Departments of Epidemiology and Public Health, and Primary Health Care.* University of Newcastle upon Tyne, Newcastle upon Tyne.

Norusis MJ (1988) *SPSS/PC+Advanced Statistics.* SPSS Inc., Chicago.

Pearson P (1992) Team work in primary health care: evaluation of a teambuilding programme. Unpublished report. Newcastle Community Health, Newcastle upon Tyne.

Poulton B and West M (1993) Effective multidisciplinary teamwork in primary health care. *Journal of Advanced Nursing* 18, 918–25.

Primary Care Clinical Audit Working Group of Clinical Outcomes Group (1994) *Clinical Audit in Primary Care,* Department of Health, London.

Spencer JA, Pearson P, James P and Southern A (1993) *Improving the Way We Work: Report of a Multi-disciplinary Audit Project.* North Tyneside Medical Audit Advisory Group, North Tyneside.

Spiegal N, Murphy E, Kinmonth AL, Ross R, Bain J and Coates R (1992) Managing change in general practice: a step-by-step guide, *British Medical Journal* 304, 231–4.

West M (1993) The reality of teamwork in primary health care. In Hearnshaw H (ed.) *Audit for Teams: The Proceedings of the Conference.* Eli Lilly National Clinical Audit Centre, Leicester.

9

Multidisciplinary clinical audit and primary health care teams

Richard Baker and Hilary Hearnshaw

Introduction

Audit, defined as the systematic critical analysis of care, was introduced for general practitioners as part of the health services reforms of 1990 (Secretaries of State for Health, Wales, Northern Ireland and Scotland, 1989). At first the emphasis was placed on audit conducted by doctors, but this policy was rapidly revised to encourage all professional groups to take part, and more recently encouragement has been given to audit undertaken by multidisciplinary teams. In this chapter we shall review the available evidence about the organisation of audit by primary health care teams, and discuss the arguments for its widespread implementation. Audit is a term that has been used to refer to a variety of related activities and, in the interests of clarity, in this chapter we shall assume that it refers to a set of activities which include the selection of a topic, the specification of desired performance in the form of review criteria and standards, collection of data about performance, the identification of deficiencies in performance compared to the standards, the implementation of improvements through the use of a range of strategies which may include one or more of education, feedback, restructured records and many others, and the collection of data for a second time in order to check that the improvements have in fact occurred.

Following the health service reforms, health authorities were required to set in place local organisations, termed medical audit advisory groups, to direct, co-ordinate and monitor audit in all local practices (Department of Health, 1990). The objective was the participation of all practices in audit. The groups were composed of local general practitioners, usually with a consultant from a local hospital, a local public health physician and occasionally a representative from health authority management. Audit groups were allowed to co-opt other members of the primary health care team with the consent of the local health authority, but initially relatively few audit groups included representatives of other professions, such as practice managers, practice or community nurses or other staff working in primary health care.

Impact of audit groups

Audit groups have been provided with financial and other resources to enable them to train general practitioners in methods of audit, and to facilitate the completion of audit projects. Therefore, because audit has required the investment of money, the impact of the audit programme has been investigated in order to determine whether the expenditure has been worthwhile. In evaluating the impact of audit groups, it is appropriate first to ask whether audit itself is an effective method for improving the quality of care. Some information which helps to answer this question can be found in a recent systematic review of good quality studies, but other reviews are being undertaken by review groups of the Cochrane Collaboration, so additional information will be available in the near future. The systematic review undertaken by Grimshaw *et al.* (1995) indicates that, whilst there is evidence from randomised controlled trials that a variety of methods can be used to implement change, no one method is always effective. Furthermore, feedback, which is often the only strategy used in audit, is less frequently effective than some other strategies, such as reminders or educational outreach. Therefore, because it is difficult to predict with confidence that a strategy to implement change will be successful, information about the impact of audit undertaken by audit groups is required.

One measure of the audit programme is the level of participation of practices. In a recent study of all 104 audit groups in England and Wales (Baker *et al.*, 1995a), the levels of participation of practices in any form of audit were reported to have risen from 71 per cent in 1991/1992 to 91 per cent in 1993/1994. In addition, audit groups had organised a large number of projects in which local practices were invited to take part. The most common topics were diabetes and asthma, but other topics explicitly included collaboration with members of the primary health care team, e.g. the involvement of practice nurses in a multidisciplinary audit of the management of patients with leg ulcers. Smaller practices are less likely to undertake audit than large ones (Jones and Dunleavey, 1992; Chambers *et al.*, 1995). The latter study also indicated that audit was more likely to be undertaken in practices which had a practice manager, raising the possibility that the presence of a team in some way facilitates audit. In a study of the reasons for non-participation in audit, smaller practices were again found to be less likely to take part, but the explanation was related to behavioural and attitudinal factors, rather than merely to practice size (Baker *et al.*, 1995b). When discussion had taken place between members of the practice, completion of the audit was more likely. Thus a basic level of teamwork may be a desirable precursor to successful audit.

As yet, there is only limited information about the impact of the audit programme on patient care. A small number of projects organised by audit groups have been reported to have improved care (Holden *et al.*, 1994; Fraser *et al.*, 1995), although examples undertaken by individual practices are relatively easy to find (Cooper *et al.*, 1994). Future studies are likely to provide more accurate information about the audit programme, but the evidence now available indicates that the organisation and methodologies of audits could be improved. The need to improve the effectiveness of audit has been recognised by the NHS Executive, and one aspect that has been singled out for improvement is greater multidisciplinary working (National Health Service Executive, 1996). Audit groups have recognised the need for greater collaborative working, and this is increasingly reflected in their membership and activities (Humphrey and Berrow, 1993). In reviewing the progress and future development of audit in primary care, a working group of the Department of Health has recommended the introduction of quality assurance which would embrace a wide range of activities, including audit, and which would be an integral part of the management of the primary health care unit (Primary Health Care Clinical Audit Working Group of Clinical Outcomes Group, 1995). In the latest restructuring of audit in primary care, encouragement has been given by the Department of Health to progress towards multidisciplinary audit (National Health Service Executive, 1995). It is now assumed that audit groups will include members of primary health care teams such as practice nurses or practice managers, and that audit will usually involve the co-operation of several professional groups. Underlying these developments is the assumption that multidisciplinary audit is, in some way, better than audit undertaken by single professional disciplines.

Investigation of the work of audit groups does indicate that they have accepted the need for multidisciplinary activity. For example, in a recent survey of audit group facilitators (Berrow *et al.*, 1996), information was sought about collaborative quality improvement projects. The 85 responding facilitators identified 188 projects that involved collaboration between different professional groups, e.g. core members of the primary health care team, community services personnel, such as specialist nurses, district nurses or social workers, and staff in other organisations, such as nursing homes, pharmacies or the ambulance service. The rapid realisation among audit groups that, in order to encourage audit in practices, primary health care teams would have to be involved, is evident from other studies of audit groups (Humphrey and Berrow, 1993, 1995), and methods of facilitating multidisciplinary audit in primary health care teams have been developed by audit group support staff (Hearnshaw *et al.*, 1994; Reddish *et al.*, 1995).

The gradual replacement of unidisciplinary by multidisciplinary audit is taking place not only in primary care, but has been promoted in secondary care as well, the overall aim being the development of a quality system for the NHS in which all professionals take part (National Health Service Management Executive, 1993a). It is envisaged that audit will also take place between different teams in collaboration across the interface between primary and secondary care. Therefore, although this chapter will consider only primary health care teams, it should be acknowledged that it is not some peculiarity of these teams that makes multidisciplinary audit appropriate to them, but rather that audit itself is viewed as being an activity that is most effective when undertaken by teams.

The nature of multidisciplinary clinical audit in primary health care

Whilst there is general consensus that multidisciplinary audit or quality assurance is a desirable goal for primary health care teams, there is less agreement about what this concept represents. Before considering how multidisciplinary audit could be introduced by primary health care teams, or what benefits, if any, might result from this, it is essential to have a clear idea of exactly what such audit entails. In this section we shall attempt to provide a classification for defining multidisciplinary audit. While we recognise that the use of evidence-based criteria, details of data collection or the completion of the audit cycle are fundamental to the effectiveness of audit, we are concentrating on the role of the primary care team. Therefore, it will be assumed that, at all stages in the development of full multidisciplinary audit, the quality of individual audits is uniformly good.

It is important from the outset to recognise that multidisciplinary audit is not an absolute which is either present or absent in a particular primary health care team, but that it is present in different teams to different extents, and also that it is present to varying degrees in the same team at different times. Furthermore, teams may progress from a primitive form of multidisciplinary audit to one that is more complex, in which case the introduction of audit can be viewed as a process taking place in stages. In the first stage, no audit is being undertaken at all, and this might be classified as Stage 0 (Table 9.1).

When audit was first introduced into primary care, it was envisaged that it would be undertaken largely by general practitioners alone. The audits that they undertook might involve colleagues in the team to a limited extent only, e.g. in collecting or providing information, or acting on changes implemented by the general practitioners as a result of the findings. This style of audit is essentially undertaken by a single health profession with assistance or co-operation from others, and might be classified as Stage 1 of multidisciplinary audit. For example, a general practitioner who undertakes an audit (including the data collection) of his or her personal management of patients with Parkinson's disease, with the assistance of members of the

Table 9.1 Stages in the development of a multidisciplinary audit in primary health care teams

Stage in development of audit	Description
Participation	
0	No audit at all
1	Audits undertaken by unidisciplinary groups
2	Some multidisciplinary projects undertaken
Management	
3	Policy on audit agreed and used by the team
4	Full multidisciplinary quality assurance

primary health care team in identifying patients, would be undertaking an audit of this type.

At the next stage in the development of multidisciplinary audit (Stage 2), a greater level of co-operation occurs. Members of the primary health care team now do more than assist a particular group in undertaking an audit of their own, but they together participate in the planning of an individual audit, jointly review the results and decide how to respond. The level of participation may vary in different teams, with more professional groups taking part in some teams than others, and the amount of discussion and joint decision-making also varying from one team to another. However, the principle that the audit requires the collaboration of professionals from different groups is the key feature that distinguishes this stage from Stage 1. To continue using Parkinson's disease as an example, relevant members of the team, such as general practitioners, practice and district nurses, and perhaps others outside the immediate team, such as an occupational therapist or a neurologist, meet together in order to reach a consensus on the criteria and standards for all aspects of care in which they are involved. They agree together the arrangements for data collection, and jointly introduce any changes required to improve care.

Two components of multidisciplinary audit can be described, namely the levels of participation by people with different professional skills and tasks, and the degree to which co-operation between these participants is managed. Stages 3 and 4 of the model are reached by teams when management of audit by the team is added to participation. It is possible, although unlikely, that the levels of management described at Stages 3 and 4 could be present with only unidisciplinary audit taking place.

In Stage 3, the collaboration has become more formalised. The team has discussed its attitude towards audit and the guidelines that it will follow in organising audit projects. There may be a document which records how the team will agree as to which topics will be selected for audit, who will be delegated to lead the audit, and the arrangements for reporting the results so that decisions can be made (Baker and Presley, 1990). In this way, audit has become an activity managed by the team, rather than an isolated activity undertaken on an occasional basis by individuals or multidisciplinary groups.

A model for audit managed by the teams has been described (Hearnshaw, 1993). The team management group first identifies problems which might be suitable for audits. Problems can be brought to the attention of the team in a number of ways. A team member may report a significant event, such as a patient complaint or an important clinical mistake. The difficulties caused by administrative procedures such as the appointment system might be raised, and the publication of new evidence-based guidelines recommending modifications to patient management policies or the invitation by the local audit group to take part in a multipractice audit of a topic of local importance might all be recognised as problems in the quality of the service which the team should consider. Team management, in whatever form it is constituted by individual teams, must prioritise problems and make plans to deal with those that are given the highest priority. During this process the team may refer to its business plan if it has agreed upon one.

Problems that are given high priority are addressed, and some of these problems will be suitable for resolving by audit. If there is a written policy for the organisation of audit, this is consulted and the audit is conducted in accordance with its stipulations. The findings of the audit are reported to team management so that the resolution of that particular problem can be monitored. In this Stage 3 model of multidisciplinary audit, the practice team has started to develop a system for improving quality, rather than merely applying a particular tool (audit) for addressing discrete topics.

The final stage of multidisciplinary audit (Stage 4) involves the full integration of audit into systems of team management, together with the use of a variety of other methods of quality improvement. In outlining the ways in which a team might manage for quality, Irvine (1990) allocated a special place to the development plan. The plan is agreed upon by the team and sets out its direction, priorities and strategies for several years to come. It was recommended that the first component of the plan should be a statement of overall purpose or 'mission', followed by provisional aims. In recent years the business plan has become an essential part of managing the fundholding practice (Pirie, 1994), and many non-fundholders also have practice development plans in one form or another. In addition to setting goals, such plans will include arrangements to measure achievement of goals. The extent to which the plans of most fundholders address quality of care as an integral component is probably limited at present, as plans for financial management, contracting, or the development of premises have generally taken precedence. Therefore, the existence of a development plan should not be equated with Stage 4 of multidisciplinary audit. Only those teams which have acknowledged in their plans the importance of quality of service, have included goals for quality improvement and have adopted specific quality improvement methods can be classified as being in Stage 4 (Edwards *et al.*, 1994).

The model of quality assurance for primary health care teams, as envisaged by the Primary Health Care Clinical Audit Working Group of Clinical Outcomes Group (1995), includes many of these features of managed quality improvement, with audit being one tool among several that are employed. The ideal team is depicted by the Working Group as having effective leadership and possessing a sense of direction, an organisational commitment to standards, professional competence, good management and collaborative working. A range of tools will be used, including development plans, guidelines and protocols, clinical audit, good quality data, effective information systems, personal performance appraisal, internal arrangements for identifying and responding to training and professional development needs, an accessible internal complaints procedure, and the resources of people and skills necessary for quality assurance. Audit should also be organised across the interface with secondary care (Eccles *et al.*, 1995). Furthermore, the team is expected to co-ordinate internal quality assurance with external elements such as professional registration, certification, accreditation schemes, quality-based contracts and performance monitoring of contracts. Teams in fundholding practices, and perhaps also some non-fundholders, would add to this list mechanisms to monitor the quality of service of providers, e.g. by regular surveys of patients who are referred to the provider, or by the review of audit data collected by the provider.

Total quality management, sometimes referred to as continuous quality improvement, represents a further development beyond integrated quality assurance, and is beginning to be adopted by a small number of teams (Oldham, 1993; Woollass, 1993). Total quality management is an approach for managing an organisation so as to improve continuously, through involving all staff in the identification, diagnosis and resolution of problems, concentration on the needs and wishes of the consumer, and the use of reliable data concerning performance (Oakland, 1993).

A number of health care organisations in the USA have adopted total quality management, and as a result of this experience it has been suggested that this approach should be introduced into the NHS (Berwick *et al.*, 1992). Starting in 1990, the Department of Health initiated a programme to introduce managed quality to 23 pilot sites in secondary or community care (National Health Service Management Executive, 1993b). An early report from this programme highlighted the need to seek patients' views, to encourage staff to respond positively to these needs, to provide systematic training for staff within a culture that encourages wide involvement, and to ensure effective communication. The need for top management and professional commitment was also demonstrated. The programme has given rise to examples of what might be achieved (National Health Service Management Executive 1994a,b). However, despite these early developments, convincing evidence to suggest that this method should be widely adopted is still awaited. Nevertheless, an emphasis on teamwork is a central feature of total quality management, and for that reason it may be particularly suitable for primary health care teams, but more relevant research is required before it could be recommended to teams.

Is multidisciplinary audit effective?

Before considering *how* multidisciplinary audit may be implemented, it is necessary to ask whether or not it *should* be implemented, in other words whether the costs and effort that would be required are likely to be justified by any resulting improvement in the quality of care. There is a reasonable body of evidence which indicates the importance of teamwork to the level of performance in many different work settings (Poulton and West, 1993), and this is considered elsewhere in this book, although improvement of aspects of teamwork does not invariably lead to improved performance (West, 1993).

However, it cannot be assumed that because good teamwork may be associated with improved performance, audit which is multidisciplinary will be more effective than audit which is not. Evidence is required so that a comparison of the relative effectiveness of multidisciplinary, unidisciplinary and no audit can be made, but the available evidence is limited. We shall first discuss findings from settings other than primary health care, and then consider the small number of studies that have been undertaken in primary health care. There have been no systematic reviews of this issue, although we do draw on two systematic reviews of related topics. A systematic review may eventually be completed either by members of the Cochrane Collaboration on Effective Professional Practice (CCEPP), or by other reviewers, although even then a definitive conclusion may not be possible because of the lack of large-scale randomised controlled trials with long follow-up periods.

Much of the argument in favour of multidisciplinary audit is drawn from quality improvement activities in commercial organisations (Peters, 1989; Martin, 1993; Oakland, 1993). In this context, good teamwork is accepted as an essential ingredient, and much of the work devoted to improving quality takes place in teams such as quality circles (Robson, 1982) or other quality improvement groups. However, on the basis of a review of total quality management failures, Walker (1992) suggests that organisations which view one method – particularly quality circles – as the sole solution to quality problems are likely to be disappointed.

Experimental studies in these settings are unusual and therefore, although the organisations that have quality-improving teamwork in one form or another may be more successful commercially, it is not possible to be absolutely certain that the benefits were caused by the teams or their degree of teamwork, rather than by some other factor. When these non-experimental, observational studies are linked to theoretical and empirical evidence about the behaviour of groups, an increasingly strong case can be made for teams that work effectively together as opposed to collections of individuals who do not co-operate. Tjosvold (1991) concludes from his review of research evidence that the involvement of team members in setting co-operative goals for the team, receiving feedback on their performance and having incentives strengthens their motivation and productivity. The most powerful factor appeared to be the development of relationships between team members, in which conflicts and frustrations can be openly discussed. The avoidance of conflicts may have short-term benefits with regard to productivity, but longer-term detrimental effects. In a health care team, the facilitation of multidisciplinary audit may provide opportunities for the team to experience the successful resolution of conflict or frustrations, as a result of agreement on changes to be implemented on the basis of findings obtained from performance data. Dickens (1994) has collated evidence concerning the characteristics of successful introduction of quality management to teams. These included good leadership and communication (which spread commitment and enthusiasm from the top down), involvement of all staff in quality issues and goal-setting, and explicit rewards for success.

Reports from the observation of health care teams reflect the lessons learned from commercial organisations. For example, in the total quality management pilot sites, communication between staff was a crucial issue (National Health Service Management Executive, 1994b). Training and management commitment were particularly important (National Health Service Management Executive, 1994a). In a study of groups of general practitioner trainers, Newton *et al.* (1992) identified similar potential obstacles to successful audits not only influencing the outcome of the audit, but also leading to missed educational opportunities. Examples from primary health care of the relationship between teamwork and quality are also easy to find. The following is a real example from a single team.

> The team included six general practitioners, four practice nurses, four district nurses and three health visitors. The district nurses had repeatedly expressed concern about the care of patients with varicose ulcers. Visiting patients at home and changing their dressings took a lot of time, and many patients seemed never to improve. The doctors felt that varicose ulcer was a chronic condition which was unresponsive to treatment, and were not interested in the topic. Eventually, after much prompting from the nurses, a simple audit was undertaken by the nurses and general practitioners. Sixteen patients were identified as having varicose ulcers, the mean duration of their ulcers being 4 years. They were all receiving regular care from both a nurse and a general practitioner, but a wide variety of treatments was being used. It was clear that treatment was not being systematically discussed or planned between the nurse and the general practitioner caring for each patient. It was agreed to institute regular discussions to develop treatment plans. At the second data collection 1 year later there had been a dramatic change. Half the patients with ulcers had recovered, and most of the remainder were improving. As a result of case discussions, a more co-ordinated and aggressive approach to treatment had been adopted, leading to a major improvement in the quality of life of this group of patients.

Experience or anecdotes of this nature may be sufficient to convince some primary health care teams to adopt multidisciplinary audit, particularly when such experience is supported by the generally observational, rather than experimental, evidence available from the world of commerce, and some theoretical and empirical information from organisational psychology. However, if the allocation of scarce resources to training and facilitation for multidisciplinary audit is to be justified, more convincing evidence is required. This should provide guidance not only on whether multidisciplinary audit is effective, but also on which method for introducing it to teams is most cost-effective. Of the studies that have been undertaken to date, most are concerned with audit at Stages 2 or 3 of the classification discussed above, and very few are concerned with Stage 4.

In a systematic review of programmes designed to improve the quality and economy of primary care, 36 evaluations were identified as fulfilling the criteria for inclusion in the review (Yano *et al.*, 1995). Most of the studies were undertaken in North America, but they addressed a wide range of aspects of care, including prevention, access, outcomes and the process of care. The most successful methods for enabling the achievement of primary care goals were computer-generated reminders, audit and feedback, methods based on social influence theory (academic detailing, expert review) and relocating the workload for specific functions, such as prevention co-ordination, to multi-disciplinary teams or team members. The studies identified did not include evaluations of the effects of facilitators or leadership training. In another systematic review of methods for altering physician performance, including both primary and secondary care (Davis *et al.*, 1995), the relative lack of effect of traditional continuing education was confirmed, and the value of reminders, outreach visits and, to a lesser extent, feedback was reaffirmed. However, the facilitation of multidisciplinary teamwork was not addressed, and this represents an important omission in the current effort to identify methods of improving clinical practice.

Implementing multidisciplinary audit in primary health care teams

Because there are several stages in multidisciplinary audit by a primary health care team, an implementation strategy may be designed either to introduce Stage 4 in a single step, or to enable teams gradually to progress from one stage to another. Each of these strategies has been used in different studies. However, in the absence of evidence as to which approach is more effective in the long term, it is not possible to recommend one of these strategies in preference to the other.

The first issue to consider is whether teams can adopt multidisciplinary audit without assistance, or whether support from outside the team should be provided, e.g. facilitation. Even in the absence of external assistance, some teams will introduce multidisciplinary audit. The process that takes place in these teams is unclear, but it is well established that some practices are more innovative than others. Teams that are larger, from practices that have been approved for vocational training of general practitioners and have practice managers, are more developed (Baker, 1992). Furthermore, it has been found that practices that had been approved for vocational training introduced more developments during a 9-year period than practices that were not approved (Baker and Thompson, 1995).

In a study of the characteristics of primary health care teams associated with innovation, Bosanquet and Leese (1986) found that younger doctors in larger partnerships were more likely to initiate innovations. However, there was an upper limit to the amount of innovation any team could manage at one time, and the level of available resources had a limiting effect (Bosanquet and Leese, 1988). Despite the reforms of the health service in the UK, some practices, particularly those in urban and inner city areas, still tended to lag behind in terms of practice structure and service provision (Leese and Bosanquet, 1995). West and Wallace (1991) undertook a study of innovation in eight health care teams, and found that the climate or attitude towards innovation among team members, and the level of team commitment and team collaboration, predicted the degree of innovation.

The importance of leadership in primary health care teams is unclear, as the issue has been largely neglected in research studies. The role of the team leader has been described by Adair (1987) as ensuring that the different needs of the task, the individual team members and the team as a whole are addressed. Clearly these factors might influence the success of attempts to introduce multidisciplinary audit, but convincing evidence for this is not available.

Given effective leadership, some teams may successfully adopt multi-disciplinary clinical audit. However, many teams do not have such leadership. Should research evidence indicate that teams should develop multidisciplinary audit, the provision of external support and encourage-ment might be justified, although information will be needed about which method is the most cost-effective. Possible methods include programmes to develop team leadership, which then takes on the task of adopting audit, or direct facilitation of the adoption of audit without any specific interventions to improve leadership. There is little information about the effectiveness of strategies to improve leadership in primary health care teams, and inter-ventions with this objective have generally sought to influence many aspects of team performance other than audit. Therefore, leadership development will not be considered further here. However, the alternative strategy of facilitation has received more attention.

Many health authorities employ facilitators to assist practice teams in developing aspects of their services (Allsop, 1990), and this method has been widely adopted by medical audit advisory groups. In a survey of audit groups conducted as early as 1992, relatively soon after their creation, it was found that more than 80 per cent of them employed one or two audit support staff (Griew and Mortlock, 1993). It has been pointed out that, with appropriate training, these staff could take on the task of facilitating multidisciplinary audit (Mortlock, 1993; Riddell, 1994).

A small number of studies suggest that facilitation is an effective strategy in primary care. The method was developed in a programme for improving health promotion services in Oxfordshire – the Oxford Prevention of Heart Attack and Stroke Project (OXCHECK) (Fullard *et al.*, 1984). In a randomised controlled trial in which three practices received the support of a facilitator and three did not, those practices that received facilitation reported improved recording of cardiovascular risk factors (Fullard *et al.*, 1987). In a trial of facilitation from the USA, which was concerned with the provision of services for cancer detection and prevention, 26 practices received the support of a facilitator plus education, 24 practices received education alone, 24 practices received facilitation alone, and a further 24 practices received no intervention (Dietrich *et al.*, 1992). Facilitators were shown to be more effective than either education alone or no intervention. In a controlled study of the management of childhood asthma, involving 12 general practices in Tayside, the effect of an audit facilitator was assessed (Bryce *et al.*, 1995). The facilitator assisted with the identification of patients and the organisation of their review, and care was improved for those patients assigned to the intervention group. In a randomised controlled trial of the implementation of guidelines for diabetes and asthma in 24 inner London general practices, practice outreach was employed (Feder *et al.*, 1995). The outreach consisted of three sessions with practice teams, the content being educational, although elements of the implementation method show similarities to those that would be used by a facilitator. Again, there were improvements in care in the intervention group.

These studies have investigated the effect of facilitation on a variety of activities of primary health care teams, but none of them has directly studied the effect on multidisciplinary audit. We have undertaken a small study to address this question (Hearnshaw *et al.*, 1994). Four teams were randomly allocated to receive the support of a facilitator, whilst four control teams received no intervention. A model of multidisciplinary audit was devised, equivalent to Stage 3 of the classification described above. A questionnaire for completion by the teams was developed from the model in order to measure the extent to which they were undertaking and managing multidisciplinary audit. The facilitator held five meetings with each primary health care team in order to instruct the teams about the methods and to take them through one or more audits (Table 9.2). One of the intervention teams dropped out, but those that completed the programme did develop their use of multidisciplinary audit. A comparison of the changes in scores using the questionnaire measure between control and intervention practices revealed statistically significant differences in favour of the intervention. However,

Table 9.2 The programme of interventions in a trial of the facilitation of multidisciplinary audit in primary health care (Hearnshaw *et al.*, 1994)

Meeting number	Content
1	Introduce concepts of audit and team; identify attitudes towards, and barriers to, team audit
2	Develop practice policy on audit – a written document about the organisation of audit by the team
3	Selection of topics for audit; development of methods for the audits; data collected before next meeting
4	Results of data collection reviewed; changes to improve care planned; second data collection planned
5	Review of second data collection to check for improvements; plans for further audits

this was a small study, and before final conclusions can be drawn about the effectiveness of facilitators in implementing multidisciplinary audit, a larger study with a longer follow-up period is required. The effect of the intervention on audit may only be a short-term one, and in judging cost-effectiveness, the need for continued support from a facilitator may have to be included in the costs.

No randomised trials of facilitation to implement Stage 4 multidisciplinary audit have yet been reported. We have developed the methods used in the study discussed above and undertaken a pilot study to investigate their feasibility (Baker *et al.*, 1995c). This study is as yet incomplete, but it is already clear that only a proportion of teams will be ready to embark on Stage 4 multidisciplinary audit. From a total of 147 practices in Leicestershire invited to take part, and over 20 practices that expressed initial interest, only six are managing to continue with the project. Because the gap between Stages 1 or 2 and Stage 4 is so great, it may not be possible for teams to make this transformation without substantial commitment and considerable external support.

Health service reform has been employed in several countries, the more common characteristics of such changes being improved management of primary health care and a degree of competition between primary care providers, to encourage teams to address quality. Those providers that wish to succeed in the new market-place will need to review their plans for quality, and it is possible that those which are eventually most successful will have implemented Stage 3 or 4 multidisciplinary audit. The health maintenance organisations (HMOs) of the USA are one example of this type of reform, and the independent practitioner associations (IPAs) in New Zealand are another. The multi-fund groups and total fundholder pilot practices in the UK are potential additional examples, although competition on the basis of quality of care is not yet a major factor in this country. It is still unclear whether structural changes of this nature have a greater impact on the use of multidisciplinary audit or on the quality of care than supportive measures such as facilitation.

Conclusions

The majority of clinical professionals in the NHS are involved in clinical audit and quality assurance, and the activity is seen as an integral component of efforts to improve the effectiveness of health care. It is widely accepted, although only on the basis of indirect evidence, that audit is more effective when it is undertaken by all those involved in providing the care concerned, i.e. multidisciplinary rather than unidisciplinary audit. In this chapter we have discussed the characteristics of multidisciplinary audit by primary health care teams, considered the evidence concerning its effectiveness in improving care, provided a classification of the different stages of multidisciplinary audit, and discussed different methods of implementing it.

If the experience of quality improvement in the commercial sector can be applied to primary health care, multidisciplinary audit may be an important development. However, a recurring theme throughout this chapter has been the limited amount of strong evidence available that would provide justification for the investment of scarce resources in introducing multidisciplinary audit to all primary health care teams. If our discussion has served to highlight an agenda for further research, it will have served its purpose.

Editors' summary

Baker and Hearnshaw have provided a clear overview of the history of multidisciplinary audit in the UK, and suggested a staged framework for its development. However, they rightly point out that multidisciplinary audit (or other quality improvement activity) is not something which is either definitely present or absent in a particular team – it will be present in different teams to different extents, and it will be present in the same team to varying degrees at different times. This must be recognised by those who seek to promote a systematic approach to quality improvement in primary care. Baker and Hearnshaw have gone on to give a clear exposition of current research on the effectiveness of multidisciplinary audit. Whilst there is wide acceptance that multidisciplinary audit is more effective than audit carried out by individual disciplines, it seems that more work is needed in this area. Finally, the authors have described current evidence concerning a range of strategies for the implementation of multidisciplinary audit in primary care, once again highlighting the need for further research. They conclude that, whatever the implementation strategy, only a relatively small proportion of primary health care teams are currently ready to undertake multidisciplinary audit which is fully integrated into team management and quality improvement, and that further research is needed before scarce resources are invested in introducing it more widely.

References

Adair J (1987) *Effective Teambuilding*, 2nd edn. Pan Books, London.

Allsop J (1990) *Changing Primary Care: the Role of Facilitators*. King's Fund Centre, London.

Baker R (1992) General practice in Gloucestershire, Avon and Somerset: explaining variations in standards. *British Journal of General Practice* 42, 415–18.

Baker R and Presley P (1990) *The Practice Audit Plan*. Severn Faculty RCGP, Bristol.

Baker R and Thompson J (1995) Innovation in general practice: is the gap between training and non-training practices getting wider? *British Journal of General Practice* 45, 297–300.

Baker R, Hearnshaw H, Cooper A, Cheater F and Robertson N (1995a) Assessing the work of medical audit advisory groups in promoting audit in general practice. *Quality in Health Care* 4, 234–9.

Baker R, Robertson N and Farooqi A (1995b) Audit in general practice: factors influencing participation. *British Medical Journal* 311, 31–4.

Baker R, Sorrie R, Reddish S, Hearnshaw H and Robertson N (1995c) The facilitation of multiprofessional clinical audit in primary health care teams – from audit to quality assurance. *Journal of Interprofessional Care* 9, 237–44.

Berrow D, Foot B and Humphrey C (1996) Working together for quality improvement. *Audit Trends* 4, 53–8.

Berwick DM, Enthoven A and Bunker JP (1992) Quality management in the NHS: the doctor's role – 1. *British Medical Journal* 304, 235–9.

Bosanquet N and Leese B (1986) Family doctors: their choice of practice strategy. *British Medical Journal* 293, 667–70.

Bosanquet N and Leese B (1988) Family doctors and innovation in general practice. *British Medical Journal* 296, 1576–80.

Bryce FP, Neville RG, Crombie IK, Clark RA and McKenzie P (1995) Controlled trial of an audit facilitator in diagnosis and treatment of childhood asthma in general practice. *British Medical Journal* 310, 838–42.

Chambers R, Bowyer S and Campbell I (1995) Audit activity and quality of completed audit projects in primary care in Staffordshire. *Quality in Health Care* 4, 178–83.

Cooper A, French D and Baker R (1994) *Illustrative Examples of Successful Audit. Research Report No. 2*. Eli Lilly National Clinical Audit Centre, Leicester.

Davis DA, Thompson MA, Oxman AD and Haynes RB (1995) Changing physician performance. A systematic review of the effect of continuing medical education strategies. *Journal of the American Medical Association* 274, 700–5.

Department of Health (1990) *Medical Audit in the Family Practitioner Services*. HC(FP)(90)8. Department of Health, London.

Dickens P (1994) *Quality and Excellence in Human Services*. Wiley, Chichester.

Dietrich AJ, O'Connor GT, Keller A, Carney PA, Levy D and Whaley FS (1992) Cancer: improving early detection and prevention. A community practice randomised trial. *British Medical Journal* 304, 687–91.

Eccles MP, Hunt J and Newton J (1995) A case study of an interface audit group. *Audit Trends* 3, 127–31.

Edwards P, Jones S and Williams S (1994) Audit as a component of planning. In Edwards P, Jones S and Williams S (eds) *Business and Health Planning for General Practice*, pp. 47–59. Radcliffe Medical Press, Oxford.

Feder G, Griffiths C, Highton C, Eldridge S, Spence M and Southgate L (1995) Do clinical guidelines introduced with practice based education improve care of asthmatic and diabetic patients? A randomised controlled trial in general practices in east London. *British Medical Journal* 311, 1473–8.

Fraser RC, Farooqi A and Sorrie R (1995) Use of vitamin B$_{12}$ in Leicestershire practices: a single topic audit led by a medical audit advisory group. *British Medical Journal* 311, 28–30.

Fullard E, Fowler G and Gray M (1984) Facilitating prevention in primary care. *British Medical Journal* 304, 687–91.

Fullard E, Fowler G and Gray M (1987) Promoting prevention in primary care: controlled trial of low-technology, low-cost approach. *British Medical Journal* 294, 1080–2.

Griew K and Mortlock M (1993) A study of MAAG organisation and function. *Audit Trends* 1, 89–93.

Grimshaw J, Freemantle N, Wallace S *et al.* (1995) Developing and implementing clinical practice guidelines. *Quality in Health Care* 4, 55–64.

Hearnshaw H (1993) The audit cycle managed by the primary health care team. *Audit Trends* 1, 7–8.

Hearnshaw HM, Baker R and Robertson N (1994) Multidisciplinary audit in primary healthcare teams: facilitation by audit support staff. *Quality in Health Care* 3, 164–8.

Holden JD, Hughes IM and Tree A (1994) Benzodiazepine prescribing and withdrawal for 3234 patients in 15 general practices. *Family Practice* 11, 358–62.

Humphrey C and Berrow D (1993) Developing role of medical audit advisory groups. *Quality in Health Care* 2, 232–8.

Humphrey C and Berrow D (1995) Promoting audit in primary care: roles and relationships of medical audit advisory groups and their managers. *Quality in Health Care* 4, 166–73.

Jones K and Dunleavey J (1992) Audit in general practice. *British Medical Journal* 304, 509.

Leese B and Bosanquet N (1995) Change in general practice and its effects on service provision in areas with different socioeconomic characteristics. *British Medical Journal* 311, 546–50.

Martin LL (1993) *Total Quality Management in Human Service Organizations. Sage Human Services Guide 67.* Sage Publications, Newbury Park.

Mortlock M (1993) Training for audit support staff. *Audit Trends* 1, 109–10.

National Health Service Executive (1995) *The New Health Authorities and the Clinical Audit Initiative.* Department of Health, Leeds.

National Health Service Executive (1996) *Promoting Clinical Effectiveness. A Framework for Action in and Through the NHS.* National Health Service Executive, Leeds.

National Health Service Management Executive (1993a) *Clinical Audit.* Department of Health, London.

National Health Service Management Executive (1993b) *The Quality Journey. A Guide to Total Quality Management in the NHS.* NHS Management Executive, London.

National Health Service Management Executive (1994a) *Quality in Action. Trafford Health Unit – a Case Study*. NHS Management Executive, London.

National Health Service Management Executive (1994b) *Quality in Action. The St Helier NHS Trust – a Case Study*. NHS Management Executive, London.

Newton J, Hutchinson A, Steen N, Russell I and Haimes E (1992) Educational potential of medical audit: observations from a study of small groups setting standards. *Quality in Health Care* 1, 256–9.

Oakland J (1993) *Total Quality Management*, 2nd edn. Butterworth-Heinemann, Oxford.

Oldham J (1993) TQM without fear. *Audit Trends* 1, 34–5.

Peters T (1989) *Thriving on Chaos. Handbook for a Management Revolution*. Pan Books, London.

Pirie A (1994) Business planning in general practice. In Pirie A and Kelly-Madden M (eds) *Fundholding. A Practice Guide*, pp. 37–46. Radcliffe Medical Press, Oxford.

Poulton B and West MA (1993) Measuring the effect of teamworking in primary health care. In Hearnshaw H (ed.) *Audit for Teams in Primary Care. Conference Proceedings*, pp. 7–12. Eli Lilly National Clinical Audit Centre, Leicester.

Primary Health Care Clinical Audit Working Group of Clinical Outcomes Group (1995) *Clinical Audit in Primary Health Care. Report to Clinical Outcomes Group*. Department of Health, London.

Reddish S, Sorrie R, Darling L, Hearnshaw H and Peddie D (1995) *Foundations for Quality Improvement: A Facilitator's Guide*. Leicestershire Medical Audit Advisory Group, Leicester.

Riddell J (1994) Audit assistants – careers and training. In Baker R (ed.) *National MAAG Delegate Day. Conference Proceedings*, pp. 26–9. Eli Lilly National Clinical Audit Centre, Leicester.

Robson M (1982) *Quality Circles. Member's Handbook*. Gower Publishing Company Ltd, Aldershot.

Secretaries of State for Health, Wales, Northern Ireland and Scotland (1989) *Working For Patients*. HMSO, London.

Tjosvold D (1991) *Team Organisation. An Enduring Competitive Advantage*. Wiley, Chichester.

Walker T (1992) Creating total quality improvement that lasts. *National Productivity Review* 11, 473–8.

West MA (1993) The reality of teamwork in primary health care. In Hearnshaw H (ed.) *Audit for Teams in Primary Care. Conference Proceedings*, pp. 13–14. Eli Lilly National Clinical Audit Centre, Leicester.

West MA and Wallace M (1991) Innovation in health care teams. *European Journal of Social Psychology* 21, 303–15.

Woollass T (1993) First steps in TQM. Part 2. *Audit Trends* 1, 128–31.

Yano EM, Fink A, Hirsch SH, Robbins AS and Rubenstein LV (1995) Helping practices reach primary care goals. Lessons from the literature. *Archives of Internal Medicine* 155, 1146–59.

10

Evaluating teambuilding

Pauline Pearson

Introduction

Working together effectively in primary health care teams is becoming increasingly important as the complexity of the tasks which face us grows. Early discharge of patients, day surgery and care management for older people all require primary care staff to work together more effectively. Teambuilding initiatives have become increasingly popular with purchasers as a mechanism both for encouraging practitioners to work together well, and for stimulating and maintaining flexibility in the face of change. However, few such initiatives have been evaluated in depth, and the issues confronting those who seek to evaluate teambuilding have not been widely discussed. This chapter explores a variety of methods for undertaking evaluation, and then goes on to discuss a range of issues arising from the work described, and lessons which can be learned from these.

Three evaluations will be discussed. The first of these looked at the outcome of an established teamwork training initiative, and semi-structured interviews were used with two practice teams. The second evaluation, described more fully in Chapter 8, was concerned with the impact of a teambuilding initiative targeted towards promoting multidisciplinary audit. A combination of practice visits, observation and postal questionnaires was used for this study, in which five practice teams were involved. The third evaluation looked at team function in relation to the introduction of organisational change. Semi-structured interviews, self-completion questionnaires and log sheets were used, and four practice teams took part.

Evaluation 1

Many people would agree with Sir Michael Drury, who in 1988 stated that, 'one thing that can be said about teamwork in general practice is that there is not a lot of it about'. How then can it be facilitated? The establishment of a joint teamwork training programme between Newcastle Family Health Services Authority (FHSA) and Newcastle Community Health offered the opportunity to explore the facilitation of primary care teamwork. The programme had been running for about 1 year before it was decided to undertake an evaluation. The intervention described below had been adapted in response to experience, and was thought to be working optimally. It was decided to evaluate the programme's impact on the next two practices to take part in the teambuilding programme. Pilot work was carried out with a third practice, which had previously been involved in the programme.

Aims

The evaluation started out with the following ambitious aims:

- to develop a grounded model of teamwork for primary health care;
- to examine the function of primary health care teams in the context of individual practitioners' own models;
- to describe a teamwork training programme;
- to compare and contrast the function of primary health care teams before and after the training programme.

However, in reality the evaluation mainly addressed the third and fourth aims, since there was not funding for time to pursue the first two aims in detail. The aims and objectives with which an evaluation starts should be realistic, and should take into account the requirements of stakeholders and resourcing.

Intervention

The training programme which formed the core of this evaluation took the form of an 'away-day'. Although initially overnight events were organised, these proved unpopular with practices, and by the beginning of the evaluation single days away from the practice base, running from 9 a.m. to 9 p.m. were the norm. Each 'away-day' took place at a comfortable local venue away from normal day-to-day distractions. The facilitator used a non-directive approach to help the primary health care team to look at an agenda of its own choosing. The day would include some work in small groups (both multidisciplinary and unidisciplinary), and some work involving the whole team. The intention was to help the team 'to improve things so that patients get a better deal and so that staff can increase their job satisfaction' (Newcastle FHSA information leaflet). The day culminated in a dinner at which team members were encouraged to continue to interact, but less formally.

Methods

It was decided to use semi-structured interviews with individual practice staff involved in the intervention. The range of individuals invited to the 'away-day' was left to the practice, so that the definition of 'primary health care team' used was 'the people invited to the day' – a definition owned by the practice decision-makers. Each participant was interviewed before and 3 months after the 'away-day'. Observation was considered, both as a means of examining team function and as an aid to description of the 'away-day', but was thought to hold too much potential threat. I was relatively well known to both practices as a colleague. A pilot study was conducted with another medium-sized practice, in order to test the interview schedule and the practicality of the proposed methods.

The next two practice teams to have a teambuilding session were taken as a convenient sample. One of these was a large practice (six partners) and one was a small one (two partners). Each practice was sent a written outline of the study, and was visited in order to discuss concerns. Nursing managers were also contacted and the study was discussed with them. All individuals were given the option to refuse to take part, or to withdraw at any time. In Practice A, 24 people were interviewed, and in Practice B, 13 people were interviewed.

Two semi-structured interviews were conducted with each individual. The first interview covered areas relating to concepts of and attitudes towards the team, how the team worked in practice, and expectations of or concerns about the 'away-day'. The following questions were included.

- Are you part of a team?
- Who is in your team?
- Day-to-day contacts – who with, how often and why?
- Who makes policy decisions?
- Give a specific example of the team working well and not working well.
- Fill in a self-completion scale addressing team function (based on Dyer, 1987).
- What are your expectations of and concerns about the 'away-day'?
- Is there anything else which you consider to be important about the team or the 'away-day'?

The second interview addressed perceptions of the 'away-day', as well as views of the team since that day, and also examined the perceived function of the team in practice over that time.

Each interview was designed to last no longer than 30 minutes in order to minimise disruption to the work of team members. The first round of interviews was completed within 2 weeks. The second round took rather longer, due to annual leave and staff shortages. Each interview was transcribed and the transcripts analysed using the constant comparative technique described by Strauss (1987). The teamwork scale was analysed separately using SPSS (Norusis, 1988). Team profiles were produced following a review of the transcripts and notes made during each interview.

Results

The findings of the study were grouped into three areas: team profiles; team function; and qualitative data. First of all, what was a team? When asked to define a primary health care team, some indicated that it was 'a group meeting together to discuss patients held in common and ways in which their needs (physical, psychological and social) might be met'. Others offered an elaborated model in which the team was perceived as a group working together over time to achieve a common goal in relation to the health of clients (individuals or communities). The varied resources of team members could be focused within this model to address the needs identified. At the first interview, of the 37 respondents, 25 individuals felt that they *were* part of a primary health care team, five felt that they were not, and seven indicated ambivalence: 'In a way – I don't have a lot to do with the running' (Receptionist).

When asked to list the members of the primary health care team, the respondents listed a wide range of individuals (see Figure 10.1 for the profile for Practice A). The only members listed by almost everyone were doctors

Member:	A	B	C	D	E	F	G	H	I	J	K	L	M	
GP	√	√	√	√	√	√	√	√	√	√	√	√	√	
Practice manager	√			√	√	√	√	√		√				
District nurse	√	√	√	√	√	√	√	√	√	√	√	√	√	
Practice nurse	√	√	√	√	√	√	√	√	√	√	√	√		
Health visitor	√	√	√	√	√	√	√	√	√	√	√	√		
Receptionists	√		√	√		√		√	√	√		√	√	
Community midwife	√		√	√	σ	√	√	√	√	√				
Social worker	√		?		σ							σ		
Community psychiatric nurse	√				σ									
Auxiliary	√							√	√		√			
Staff nurse	√													
Dietitian							√					σ		
Cleaner								√						
Speech therapist													σ	
Physiotherapist													σ	

Key: ? = unsure if still involved; σ = some contact.

Figure 10.1 Members of the PHCT, Practice A

and district nurses (one omission of each in practice B). Hutchinson and Gordon (1992) have commented that some respondents to their question-naire forgot to include themselves (assuming that they regarded themselves as part of the team). In this study, some roles were omitted because they were not differentiated (e.g. the secretary was not differentiated from receptionists in Practice B), and others were omitted because they had no functional contact (e.g. the community psychiatric nurse or the dietitian in Practice A).

Profiles were also drawn up on an individual level for each respondent, showing their contacts rated in one of three ways – daily or more frequently, more than weekly but not daily, and weekly or less often. The qualitative data obtained provided information about the nature of the contacts and the reasons for them. Figure 10.2 shows that two GPs from the same practice had differing profiles with regard to both the component professionals to whom they related and the frequency of interaction. It seems that function often defines team boundaries according to professional group (e.g. doctor, district nurse) or specific clinical responsibility (e.g. diabetes or child health). Some individuals identified people as having been historically part of the team. The social worker was listed in this way by one member of Practice A (see Figure 10.1). Those individuals who made such comments were relatively few, but had been in post for lengthy periods.

A second, related area for attention is the question of 'teams within teams'. This is illustrated in Figure 10.3 by two district nurses (a and b) from different practices. The day-to-day team for each nurse includes district nursing colleagues, a staff nurse or district enrolled nurse and – mentioned by only one nurse – an auxiliary. District nurse b has not mentioned the auxiliary in her practice, although she clearly interacts with her at least twice a week in an informal meeting about patients (I was present at one such meeting). Only a few other respondents in either practice mentioned that there was more than one level within the district nursing team. Thus there is a problem for some individuals of visibility within the wider team.

Some members were not only invisible, but more isolated within teams. Figure 10.4 compares the profiles for two receptionists (a and b) within one practice. Receptionist b is almost immediately identifiable as an evening receptionist by her very restricted team profile. Her day-time colleague (receptionist a) has a much fuller profile in terms of both component profes-sionals and frequency of contact. Thus, work patterns can contribute both to isolation within the team, and to more limited perceptions of its breadth.

Time in post can also contribute to skewed perceptions. A practice nurse who had only been in post for 4 weeks at the time of the initial interview had a very wide and frequent set of contacts following her induction programme. At the subsequent interview, almost 4 months later, the frequency of her contacts had decreased, and some individuals had ceased to be included.

Following the 'away-day' intervention, there was little quantitative change for most participants. However, they did identify generally positive changes in the nature of the contacts made:

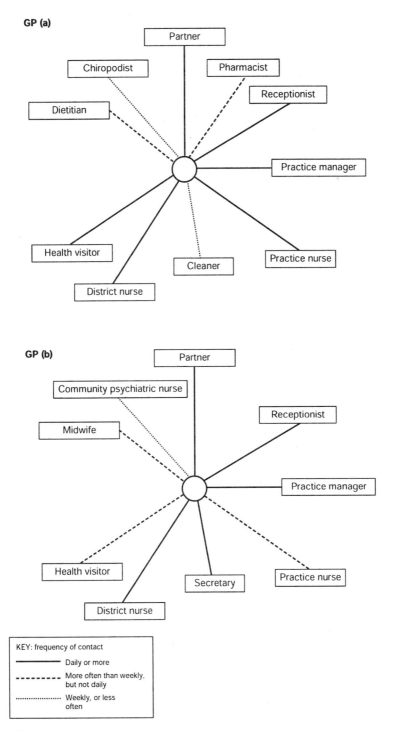

Figure 10.2

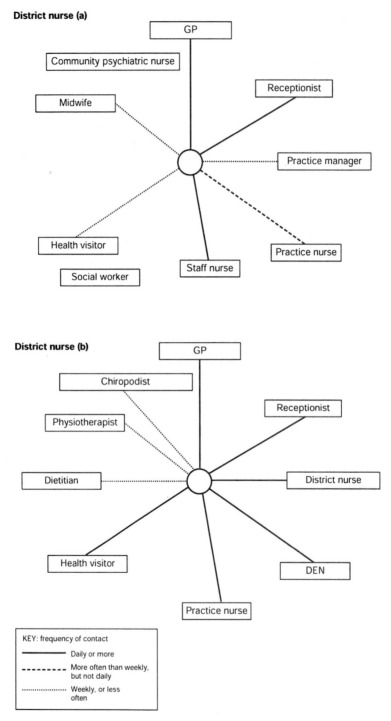

Figure 10.3

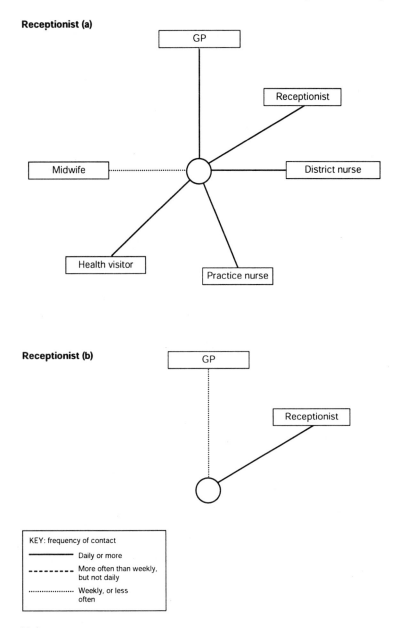

Figure 10.4

Some staff are more confident. The reception staff are more expressive. It's hard to compare, but I think even the nursing staff are more confident.

(GP)

It's easier to talk to the rest of the team. Our problems are echoed by others.

(Receptionist)

We got to know some team members better and vice versa. Things are a lot easier – you can approach issues better. . . . We say hello to one another more – there's a definite increase in that. . . . I'm more at ease going into reception and approaching people to do things.

(Health visitor)

The monthly practice meeting has evolved from the day, so that's better. . . . I find the doctors phone me at [base] more than they did before too.

(Midwife)

Team function was addressed by the administration, within the interview, of a self-completion scale modified from that developed by Dyer (1987). It consisted of nine items, with modifications to the text for a UK health professional sample. Each item was scored on a 5-point scale, with variation in direction to avoid response bias. An additional question asked respondents to score their perception of their team's delivery of health care on a similar 5-point scale derived from work by Wise *et al.* (1974). Thus 10 items were analysed (see Figure 10.5).

A	To what extent do I feel a real part of the team?
B	How safe is it in this team to be at ease, relaxed and myself?
C	To what extent do I feel 'under cover', that is, have private thoughts, unspoken reservations or unexpressed feelings and opinions that I have not felt comfortable bringing out into the open?
D	How effective are we, in our team, in getting out and using the ideas, opinions and information of all team members in making decisions?
E	To what extent are the goals the team is working towards understood, and to what extent do they have meaning for me?
F	How well does the team work at its tasks?
G	Our planning and the way we operate as a team are largely influenced by . . .
H	What is the level of responsibility for work in our team?
I	How are differences and conflicts handled in our team?
X	Where do we feel our team is at present (in terms of health care delivery)?

Figure 10.5 Items included in teamwork scale

The items were first examined in order to determine whether there was any significant difference between the scores at the first and second interviews – in other words, any difference potentially attributable to the 'away-day'. Of the 10 items examined, eight showed a change in score, suggesting an improvement in aspects of team functioning. Four of these shifts in score – for items C, D, E and X – were found to be significantly different between the interviews when a t-test was carried out. The two items which did not show any improvement related to how well the team was seen to work at its tasks, and the level of responsibility taken for work in the team. Further analysis was performed in order to examine the differences between the first and second interviews for different employment groups, namely attached staff, employed staff and doctors. The results of this analysis suggested that the greatest effect was on attached staff, and the least on doctors. However, the number of doctors was small, so caution must be exercised when interpreting the data for them.

A substantial proportion of the data collected in the interviews was qualitative. The questions explored day-to-day functioning, perceived strengths and weaknesses of team functioning (seeking to focus on critical incidents) and expectations or perceived outcomes of the intervention. The interviews were transcribed and were then analysed using constant comparative analysis (Strauss, 1987). Seven key concepts emerged.

Communication

This was a central concept in respondents' discussion of their relationship with other team members, and in descriptions of 'good' or 'bad' teamwork. Respondents highlighted 'passing messages' and having time to communicate as themes.

Getting to know people

Getting to know one another, and valuing team members as people, were clearly important from the earliest transcripts. After the 'away-day', many individuals commented that other team members were more approachable than they had been previously. Some said that they consciously tried to remember team members with whom they had less contact. Systems were developed which even helped part-time staff.

Hierarchies

Some respondents talked about hierarchies, while others discussed the importance of autonomy. Hierarchies were generally perceived as having been reduced following the 'away-day': 'You don't always feel it's the doctors in control' (Practice manager). However, for some it was still hard to 'all be equal for the day' (Receptionist).

Difficult team members

Common to both teams and to many of the respondents was the idea of someone (usually unspecified) within the team who presented problems – a difficult team member. Each team had at least one of these. Even after the 'away-day' this problem was not resolved. Training in this area was felt to be potentially valuable.

Isolation

Another recurring theme was that of isolation: 'We meet but I feel we work in isolation' (Health visitor). Certain groups appeared to feel particularly isolated, namely receptionists and health visitors, although the reasons for this were not clear.

Acknowledgement

Acknowledgement of the roles played by individuals was another area highlighted by some team members, particularly those who felt that their role was poorly understood, namely auxiliaries and reception staff. Improvements following the 'away-day' were described in terms of being valued and acknowledged: 'It's a good feeling to know you're listened to' (Auxiliary).

Effective practice

Respondents were asked prior to the 'away-day' to identify changes which they would like to see take place in practice, reflecting better teamwork. Most of the changes that were identified related to improvements in communication, but some were directly beneficial to patients, e.g. moving furniture to ensure privacy for patients at reception.

Specific comments about the 'away-day' were also examined. Three descriptions predominated: 'useful', 'enjoyable' and 'hard work'. Positive comments reflected many of the concepts highlighted above, i.e. getting to know one another, having time to communicate, sharing ideas and identifying problems. Negative comments were few, but those that were made stressed the need to deal with difficult team members, and the hard work involved in participating.

Evaluation 2

The second evaluation is described more fully in Chapter 8. It formed part of an intervention targeted at promoting multidisciplinary audit, based in North Tyneside, a borough bordering Newcastle. This involved the provision of two teambuilding half days for each participating team, together with information on developing and implementing an audit plan, and access to specialist assistance. The evaluation was concerned to measure the impact of the overall initiative, including the teambuilding sessions. A combination of practice visits, observation and postal questionnaires was used for this study, in which five practice teams were involved. The aims of the evaluation were as follows:

- to describe the intervention used;
- to compare and contrast the multidisciplinary audit activity of primary health care teams before and after the training programme.

Intervention

The intervention was facilitated in a similar manner to the sessions described above. Each half-day session took place at a venue removed from normal day-to-day distractions. The facilitator used a non-directive approach to help the primary health care team to look first at its own functioning and then at issues which might require auditing. The team was then encouraged to review its functioning and to examine its progress in relation to its audit plan.

Methods

As with the Newcastle study, the range of individuals invited to participate was decided by the practices themselves. Although the pattern of data collection was broadly similar to the Newcastle study, for reasons of resourcing and a tight time scale it was not feasible to interview all of the participants – with five practices there were large numbers of staff to include. All of the practices were visited three times by the intervention team and evaluator. However, each individual was then sent a postal questionnaire immediately before and about 2 weeks after completion of the intervention. The questionnaire was similar to the interview schedule described above, but included a number of questions designed to ascertain participants' views on and knowledge of audit. The teams were also invited to two evening meetings in order to share information about progress, and teambuilding sessions were observed. Finally, each practice was asked to produce a progress report at the end of the study period. Analysis combined thematic analysis of questionnaires, visit notes and observation data with the use of descriptive statistics and *t*-tests on scale data.

Differences

Most of the findings of this evaluation are reported in Chapter 8. Here I shall comment on the areas in which this study differed from its predecessor. First, the overall response rate was lower than that in the Newcastle study. In

Newcastle, the initial response rate was 91 per cent. The response rate for the second interview fell to 86 per cent. In North Tyneside, the initial response was similar (94 per cent), but the response to the second round of questionnaires fell to 65 per cent. This may have been because the interviews involved specially booked time, whilst the questionnaires could be continually put off until later. The literature suggests that studies employing interviews normally show a better response rate (Oppenheim, 1992). Another possible explanation is that I was known to most of the Newcastle participants, whereas I was unknown to the majority of staff in the North Tyneside practices.

Secondly, although some significant overall improvements were observed in the results obtained on Dyer's modified scale (for the categories related to understanding the team's goals and influencing planning), with this sample the changes categorised according to staff group were not consistent. However, with the larger number of teams involved, analysis could also be undertaken by practice. This showed that all but one of the practices made improvements in most areas, and the practices that scored most highly at the start (i.e. which were functioning best) continued to do well.

Thirdly, observation was used in this study. I recorded how individuals and small groups interacted during the interventions, sketching seating arrangements and mapping interactions within groups to see if any patterns appeared, and I reflected on possible reasons for these behaviours. Written notes were analysed thematically, comments grouped and the interaction maps annotated. However, whilst observation was useful in enabling me to describe the intervention, few of the data appeared to be helpful in answering the main evaluation question – whether the intervention produced any change in the practice teams' capacity to work together at audit.

Evaluation 3

The third evaluation took place in Northumberland, and examined team function in relation to the introduction of organisational change. Nurses were felt to be poorly integrated into primary health care decision-making. It was decided to test the idea of a 'team management executive' combining a nursing representative, a doctor and an administrative representative. The aims of the evaluation were as follows:

- to describe the process of introducing the executives;
- to examine the functioning of the primary health care teams before and after the introduction of the executives;
- to investigate purchasers' and providers' perceptions of the executives.

Intervention

Each team management executive consisted of members elected to provide a nursing representative, a doctor and an administrative representative. The nurses elected in each case were attached staff, and the administrative representatives were the practice managers. The executive was responsible for negotiating contracts in relation to nursing involvement in the team and for developing specific clinical protocols. The participating practices had all recently taken part in a teambuilding exercise, and were considered anecdotally to be functioning well. One practice was fundholding, two practices had formed a consortium and were 'shadow fundholders', and the remaining practice was not intending to become fundholding.

Methods

The evaluation was performed for the Health Authority by Lesley Duke, a senior registrar in public health, and I acted as supervisor for the project. Staff in each practice, FHSA staff members and community nursing managers were interviewed soon after the beginning of the project, using semi-structured interviews, to determine their views of the scheme. Self-completion questionnaires incorporating Dyer's team functioning scale were issued after the team executive had existed for 6 months, in order to identify levels of team functioning. From the start of the project, log sheets were issued and members were asked to record examples of positive and negative effects of involvement in the management executive pilot as they occurred. Log sheets were collected fortnightly during the evaluation period by a research assistant working with Dr Duke, and 50 per cent of all log sheets were collected in the first 10 weeks; returns were regular but slow thereafter. A total of 180 comments were collected. Interviews and log sheets were subjected to thematic analysis, and scale data were analysed using descriptive statistics and *t*-tests.

Differences

The results of this study have been reported elsewhere (Duke, 1994). Here I shall focus on the areas in which this study differed from the others discussed above. First, there was no specific teambuilding intervention during the project, although all of the teams had recently participated in one. The intervention was instead specifically intended to alter the decision-making within the primary health care team, especially in relation to the nursing component. The Dyer scale was used only once, due to delays in operationalising the evaluation. However, the team which had the highest overall scores on this scale also showed the greatest positive impact on decision-making in the qualitative results.

Secondly, log sheets were used to identify examples of positive and negative effects of the pilot scheme as they occurred. Rather than relying upon individual recall in interviews or questionnaires, data were collected contemporaneously. Although some difficulty was experienced in persuading staff to contribute as time went on, a substantial database was generated of events that individuals felt illustrated positive or negative aspects of the scheme. Recurring topics included positive comments about communication and developments arising and negative comments about the time involved and the emotions stirred up. As a mechanism for collecting illustrations of the practical experience of individuals underlying the relatively superficial assessment contained in Dyer's scale, log sheets appear to be satisfactory.

Issues in evaluation

Evaluation is a complex task, akin to research, but often requiring more pragmatic solutions to methodological dilemmas. It must seek to answer six questions in relation to any intervention.

- What is the context of the intervention?
- What is the intervention process?
- What is the outcome of the intervention (i.e. is it effective)?
- Is the intervention acceptable?
- Is the intervention efficient?
- Is the intervention cost-effective?

Some of these questions are more important than others to different stakeholders. The evaluation should focus on the stakeholders' priorities (see Chapters 13 and 14). A number of methodological issues arise from the studies described here, and these are discussed below.

Sampling and variability

One of the common problems in evaluative research is the restricted nature of sampling. In the Newcastle evaluation, a convenience sample was used, namely the next two practices to undergo 'teambuilding'. As it happened, these were two quite different practices with similar outcomes. However, it is clear from North Tyneside that the more practices that are involved, the greater is the potential for variability in team profiles, team functioning and perceptions of teamworking. Should more practices have been involved in Newcastle? Inclusion of the next practice involved would have led to a delay of 9 months in delivery of the evaluation report. Another criticism which could be made of all three evaluations is that the practices sampled were those willing to co-operate, so they were perhaps not representative of run-of-the-mill primary health care. This will always tend to be the case, since the practices that fail to co-operate are likely to be those who see least value in change. Although the practices included in the evaluations varied widely, from large fundholding group practices with extensive teaching commitments to a small single-handed practice with limited potential for development, there is scope for larger studies to attempt to involve more 'ordinary' practices.

Choosing methods – options and intentions

The choice of methods must depend in part on the problem to be addressed, and in part on the context in which the evaluation occurs. In each of these evaluations slightly different methods were employed. In Newcastle, interviews were decided upon as the primary method of data collection. Although they can be labour-intensive, the time required for two practices was resourced adequately. The pay-off is in the higher quality of data obtained, and the response rate. In North Tyneside, questionnaires were used because of the numbers of staff to be included in the data collection. These were simpler to administer, but produced lower response rates. Use of the Dyer scale with more groups highlighted its potential for showing variability *between* teams. However, it has not been validated against other measures so as to demonstrate whether this variability is real or an artefact of organisational arrangements. The scale was designed for use across the same team over time, and appears to be satisfactory in identifying perceived changes in functioning in this context. In Northumberland, the Dyer scale was used only once, and when only one aspect of team functioning was the subject of the intervention, namely decision-making. In this context, even if it had been repeated, one would not have expected statistically significant changes to be recorded. However, supplementing the scale with qualitative data from interviews and log sheets allowed specific aspects of team functioning to be explored in more depth. Log sheets in particular enabled the collection of illustrations of the practical experience of individuals to flesh out the outline contained in Dyer's scale.

Time and ownership

In the primary care setting, time is of importance to both the researcher and those being researched. The busy GP or nurse will not co-operate with a study which does not take account of his or her schedule. Staff may be unwilling to give up their own time for an evaluation, particularly if they will not be the main beneficiaries. The Newcastle and Northumberland studies were joint initiatives between purchasers and providers, with no obvious pay-off for the practices themselves. Feedback was given to one practice meeting, and was given in written form to others. However, feedback can be a mixed blessing in promoting co-operation, since people worry about attribution. The North Tyneside study was the result of a bid by the local Medical Audit Advisory Group (MAAG), of which GPs from three of the five practices involved were members. It could therefore be argued that they saw some benefit in the study. However, this was not the case for all of the teams involved.

Attribution issues

Attribution is a problem for people in most evaluations – they are concerned lest the comments that they may make about the project, its functioning or the individuals involved may be attributed to them. In other words, will what they say be confidential? Where feedback is offered to participants, such concerns are particularly strong. Assurances of confidentiality may be mistrusted. In general, people in Newcastle appeared to be willing to share their feelings with me. I was known to most of them, and may have benefited from their previous experience of me. In North Tyneside the questionnaire was anonymous. Individuals might still feel that their responses were identifiable, if for example they were the only receptionist working on the diabetic clinic, or the only GP with an interest in the health of the elderly. However, the response rate was still satisfactory. I was not well known to them, but the evaluation was closely associated with the University, and colleagues of high standing. The MAAG's involvement with the project may also have facilitated its acceptability. In North Tyneside and Northumberland, the evaluation was part of the programme on offer. However, there was some evidence in the patterns of refusal in both evaluations that GPs felt less apprehensive about participation than other groups.

Presentation

In evaluation, the way in which findings are presented is particularly important. The results are usually destined to be used in decisions about the continuation of an intervention or project. In order to influence policy, the results must be readily understood. Three specific issues arise in these evaluations. First, data such as the score on Dyer's scale can be presented in a number of ways. In Newcastle, the data were presented verbally and in tabular form. In North Tyneside, they were presented graphically. On balance, the latter format appeared to be more accessible to practice staff reading the report.

Secondly, data such as team profiles for individuals need to be presented in a way that is easily understood, and not too 'busy' or detailed. Readers' understanding of the data can be enhanced if key issues are clearly illustrated, as in Figures 10.2, 10.3 and 10.4. Detailed profiles were appended to the original Newcastle report, in order to avoid overloading the reader.

Thirdly, qualitative data formed a significant part of each of these studies. The way in which qualitative data are reported has been recognised as an important factor in determining the way in which they are used (Melia, 1987). Different approaches were taken in these studies. In the Newcastle study, qualitative material was reported as a series of concepts derived from the data. Time constraints prevented the development of a theoretical framework describing the interrelationships of these concepts. In the

Northumberland study, log diaries provided illustrations of the experience of individual team members. These were grouped and used to discuss the various aspects of decision-making within the report.

Influencing policy

As well as ensuring that the results are presented in such a way that they can be readily understood, evaluations will not influence policy unless they are timely and address the right questions. Although the first evaluation was delivered within the agreed time scale, and indicated that the intervention produced a significant change in team functioning, it did not facilitate the continuation of the teambuilding programme, which ceased about 1 year after the report. The evaluation was not timely, nor did it address the right questions. It was commissioned in 1991, at a time when increasing political emphasis was being placed on team effectiveness and efficiency. Although it improved on evaluations which had largely examined 'happiness' with teambuilding (Spratley, 1989; see Chapter 6), it was still restricted to examining whether the intervention could be associated with changes in aspects of each team's functional process. Whilst a few years earlier such an evaluation would have been regarded as valuable, at this point it did not answer the commissioners' questions. At the time when it was commissioned, neither I nor the appointed steering group realised the importance of looking at effectiveness. Furthermore, although costs were examined, they were not weighted adequately by measures of benefit. The lesson is to consider not only the explicit questions asked, but also the policy shifts within which the intervention occurs, in order to identify the implicit questions. Above all, the six key questions listed above must each be carefully reflected upon.

Resourcing

Resources have been alluded to on a number of occasions, and resources may include time, or money to pay for time, or indeed equipment to facilitate the use of time. In Newcastle, insufficient time led to restrictions on the level of analysis that could be achieved. This was partly due to underestimation at the point of design, but was also caused by competing demands on me as the sole evaluator. In North Tyneside, with substantially more participants, the resources were only sufficient to permit the issue of questionnaires to participants. Funding for an assistant, or greater time commitment from me, were not feasible. The impact of this has been described above. In Northumberland, the design of the evaluation was constrained by lack of time to gather adequate baseline data. The intervention was almost in place when the evaluation was considered and an evaluator appointed. This problem is frequently encountered in evaluation (see also Chapter 14), and may also result in hasty and perhaps inadequate design. Resources were available to employ a research assistant to collect more detailed data at a later stage. Whilst this did not compensate for problems in identifying change, both process and outcome were well described.

Conclusions

This chapter has looked at three evaluations of teamwork and teambuilding, using a variety of approaches. A number of issues have been highlighted by these evaluations, including the importance of sampling and the potential for variability, the potential of different methods for answering specific questions, issues related to time and ownership, questions about attribution and confidentiality, the importance of presentation, timing and appropriateness in influencing policy and, last but not least, resource issues. Overall, the clearest message must be that the design of any evaluation of teambuilding or teamwork must be well thought out, and must address the key evaluation questions. Furthermore, where resources, whether these be time, manpower or equipment, are limited it must be recognised that this is likely to restrict the depth and quality of the evaluation.

Editors' summary

This chapter has provided a very practical overview of evaluative research on teambuilding. Pearson has looked at some of the methods which can be used and the issues arising in the evaluation of teambuilding initiatives. She has described the use of interviews, questionnaires, log sheets or diaries and observation, highlighting the strengths and weaknesses of each. The methodological issues discussed include problems with sampling, difficulties in choosing and using methods, the importance of presenting results appropriately, issues arising in seeking to influence policy, and limitations imposed by restricted resources.

References

Duke L (1994) *Primary Care and Community Nursing. Pilot Report to Health Authority.* Northumberland Health Authority, Morpeth.

Dyer W (1987) *Teambuilding: Issues and Alternatives.* Addison-Wesley, Reading, MA.

Hutchinson A and Gordon S (1992) Primary care teamwork: making it a reality. *Journal of Interprofessional Care* 6, 31–42.

Melia K (1987) *Learning and Working: the Occupational Socialization of Nurses.* Tavistock Publications, London.

Norusis M J (1988) *The SPSS Guide to Data Analysis for SPSS.* SPSS Inc., Chicago.

Oppenheim A (1992) *Questionnaire Design, Interviewing and Attitude Measurement,* 2nd edn. Pinter, London.

Spratley J (1989) *Disease Prevention and Health Promotion in Primary Health Care*. Health Education Authority, London.

Strauss A (1987) *Qualitative Analysis for Social Scientists*. Cambridge University Press, Cambridge.

Wise H, Beckhard R, Rubin I and Kyte A (1974) *Making Health Teams Work*. Ballinger, Cambridge, MA.

Acknowledgements

Thanks are due to John Spencer and Alice Southern for their reflections on the North Tyneside evaluation, and to Lesley Duke for allowing me to include details of her Northumberland study.

11

Defining and measuring effectiveness for primary health care teams

Brenda Poulton and Michael West

Introduction

Since the instigation of the NHS in 1948 the health needs of British society have changed. We now have an increasingly elderly population resulting in more chronic disease, and the most prevalent diseases are lifestyle related (e.g. coronary heart disease). These changes have resulted in a shift in focus for primary health care from simple diagnosis and treatment, to include health promotion and chronic disease management. These new priorities were articulated in the White Paper *Promoting Better Health* (Department of Health and Social Security, 1987), subsequently enacted through the 1990 GP Contract (Health Departments of Great Britain, 1989). The contract placed greater emphasis on health promotion by introducing target payments for health screening and immunisation. These extended responsibilities have resulted in a broader range of skills being required for primary health care delivery, and subsequent expansion of the size of primary health care teams (Audit Commission, 1993).

The concept of the primary health care team has been around for several decades and is repeatedly recommended in several reports (Department of Health and Social Security, 1981; Department of Health and Social Security, 1986; National Health Service Management Executive, 1993). One of the most recent contributions to the debate is an innovative report which examines nursing in primary care (National Health Service Management Executive, 1993) and states:

> The best and most cost-effective outcomes for patients and clients are achieved when professionals work together, learn together, engage in clinical audit of outcomes together, and generate innovation to ensure progress in practice and service.
>
> (paragraph 4.3)

However, there is evidence to suggest that teamwork among doctors, nurses and administrators in primary health care is more rhetoric than reality (Bond *et al.*, 1985). A recent Audit Commission Report (1992) summarises some of the problems of multidisciplinary teamwork in primary health care as follows:

> Separate lines of control, different payment systems leading to suspicion over motives, diverse objectives, professional barriers and perceived inequalities in status, all play a part in limiting the potential of multi-professional, multi-agency teamwork. These undercurrents often lead to rigidity within teams, with members adhering to narrow definitions of their roles, preventing the creative and flexible responses required to meet a variety of human need presented. They are also likely to lower morale. For those working under such circumstances efficient teamwork remains elusive.
>
> (Audit Commission, 1992, p. 20)

Against this background we carried out a study to explore teamworking in primary care and to relate it to effectiveness of outcomes (Poulton, 1995). The initial research question posed was as follows. What factors make a primary health care team (PHCT) work well as a team, and can these factors be measured?

This led on to two further questions.

- Are PHCTs that work well as teams more effective?
- How do we conceptualise and measure effectiveness for PHCTs?

Developing measures of teamworking and PHCT effectiveness

A review of the organisational psychology literature (Poulton, 1995) demonstrated that the input–process–output model dominates much of the most recent research. The following key themes emerged from the empirical evidence as influencing work group effectiveness:

- team structures;
- team interaction processes;
- the nature of the team task;
- team norms;
- team goals;
- performance feedback;
- the organisational context in which the team operates.

These themes were used as a basis for the measures developed in the research.

Prior to our study, no research on the factors predicting effectiveness in PHCTs had been undertaken, and it was therefore difficult to select the most appropriate empirical framework for the exploration of PHCT effectiveness. Indeed, the complex issue of what constitutes PHCT effectiveness had never been addressed. It seemed, therefore, that the input–process–output framework presented the soundest option, given that it is the most empirically tested model. In addition, in terms of health care, the structure–process–outcome configuration is a familiar model in the field of quality assurance (Donabedian, 1966, 1980).

To simplify the approach, it was decided to include team structures and how these were organised as inputs. Team interaction processes, norms and goals were included as process aspects, and finally the consequences of team activities are the outputs.

Input and process variables were measured by means of the Primary Health Care Team Questionnaire (PHCTQ), the bulk of which was composed of the Team Climate Inventory (Anderson and West, 1994). Output variables were measured by means of the Primary Health Care Team Effectiveness Questionnaire (PHCTEQ).

Measuring teamwork: inputs and processes

To address the input and process aspects of the conceptual model, we administered the PHCTQ to all members of the 68 PHCTs in the study described on page 19. Respondents were asked to complete the questionnaire anonymously and to return it directly to the researchers in a prepaid envelope. The questionnaire was divided into seven sections. Section 1 collected information on biographical aspects of the respondent, and these constituted the input factors of the model. It asked members of the team to state:

- their job title;
- the number of people in their team;
- how long they had worked in the team;
- whether the practice was fundholding.

Sections 2 to 5 consisted of the four team climate factors based on the Team Climate Inventory (Anderson and West, 1994), which measured four elements of team functioning, namely participation, shared objectives, task orientation and support for innovation. These elements are discussed in detail in Chapter 2.

Section 6 incorporated three measures of role understanding and valuing, and Section 7 asked respondents to state their personal perception of their team's objectives and provided space for any further comments they wished to make about their team. The remaining sections of the PHCTQ measured team process factors. We provide more detailed information about the scales used to measure team process factors below.

Participation

This scale consisted of 12 items designed to measure participation in the team. Eight of the items related directly to participation, for example:

We share information generally in the team, rather than keeping it to ourselves.

People feel understood and accepted by each other.

Four of the items related to interaction in the team, for example:

We interact frequently.

Members of the team meet frequently to talk both formally and informally.

Respondents were asked to rate each of the items on a scale of 1 (strongly disagree) to 5 (strongly agree).

Shared objectives

This part of the questionnaire used an 11-item scale relating to team objectives. For example:

How clear are you about what your team's objectives are?

To what extent do you think they are useful and appropriate objectives?

Respondents were asked to rate statements on a scale of 1 (not at all) to 7 (completely).

At the end of the questionnaire, respondents were asked to state their team's objectives.

Task orientation

For the purpose of this study a 7-item scale relating to task performance was used. For example:

Do you and your colleagues monitor each other so as to maintain a higher standard of work?

Does the team critically appraise potential weaknesses in what it is doing in order to achieve the best possible outcomes?

Respondents were asked to rate their team on a scale of 1 (not at all) to 7 (completely).

Support for innovation

The questionnaire used an 8-item scale to measure support for new ideas. For example:

This team is open and responsive to change.

Team members provide practical support for new ideas and their application.

Respondents were asked to rate items on a scale of 1 (strongly disagree) to 5 (strongly agree).

Mutual role understanding

The importance of team roles in the achievement of tasks is a recurring theme within the organisational psychology literature (Hackman and Morris, 1975; Sundstrom *et al.*, 1990; Guzzo and Shea, 1992). There is an emphasis on the fact that the right mix of roles should be available to provide necessary skills for the task to be achieved. There is also an assumption that roles should be flexible and evolve in response to change. In contrast to such philosophies, it has been shown that roles and skills within PHCTs are not determined by need (Lightfoot *et al.*, 1992), and that there is a high degree of role protection and role misunderstanding among various members of the PHCT (Department of Health and Social Security, 1981, 1986; Bond *et al.*, 1985; Audit Commission, 1992). Consequently, it is assumed that teamwork will be more effective if individual team members are clear about their own roles, and understand and value the roles of their fellow team members (Department of Health and Social Security, 1981).

The following three questions were therefore included in the PHCTQ in order to tap these elements of role valuing and understanding.

- 'Please indicate the extent to which, on average, the different groups in your practice (e.g. doctors, nurses, receptionists) make appropriate use of your skills . . . . In our practice they make appropriate use of my skills . . .'
- 'Please indicate the extent to which, on average, you know and understand the roles of different groups in your practice (e.g. doctors, nurses, receptionists) . . . . I understand what areas of knowledge are required in their role in our practice . . .'
- 'Please indicate your attitudes towards the roles of other groups in your practice team. . . . I consider this role vital in the achievement of team objectives.'

For each statement, respondents were given a list of core team members (district nurses, GPs, health visitors, practice manager, practice nurses, receptionists) plus others (to be specified). They were asked to rate the statement in relation to each practitioner on a scale of 1 (not at all) to 5 (completely).

In order to confirm the structure of the scales, the data collected in the study were subjected to factor analysis, which is a method of grouping data to make them easier to analyse. In this procedure, groups of items are correlated and examined in relation to specific factors, and a scale is then developed for each dimension of the concept being measured. The factor analysis confirmed the four-factor structure for the team climate factors demonstrated by Anderson and West (1994). The role understanding variables were related to three factors which confirmed the conceptual model, namely appropriate skill use, knowledge of fellow team member roles, and valuing of individual roles. In order to establish whether each scale measured a single item and thus to determine whether the items that constitute the scale were internally consistent, we calculated Cronbach's alpha coefficient for each of the scales. For a comprehensive description of the calculation and interpretation of Cronbach's alpha, see Bryman and Cramer (1990). All of the scales displayed acceptable levels of internal reliability as indicated by Cronbach's alpha test (Poulton, 1995).

Measuring primary health care team effectiveness: outputs

Within any assessment of effectiveness there are a number of stakeholders (Connally *et al.*, 1980), all of whom might use different criteria to judge effectiveness. PHCTs exist to maintain and improve the health of their populations through health promotion, treatment and rehabilitation. Patients and their carers are therefore major stakeholders in this process but, as much of their care is provided free at the point of service, the allocation and management of resources rests with other stakeholders, notably health commissioners and providers. These major groups of stakeholders will have conflicting criteria for effectiveness – patients and carers want to be given high-quality care which may be costly, whereas health commissioners and providers need to deliver the necessary care within allocated resources.

In order to develop measures of effectiveness that incorporate the views of all stakeholders, we convened a seminar to which we invited representatives from all stakeholder groups, ranging from patients and carers to providers and commissioners, to NHS Executive representatives. As a result of this seminar we generated a large number of effectiveness criteria (Poulton and West, 1994). These criteria were incorporated into a questionnaire which was piloted with 245 practice nurses (Poulton and West, 1996a) and subsequently amended to form the PHCTEQ. The questionnaire covers the following four broad areas.

- Patient satisfaction with services related to the quality of patient information, the continuity of care, and the empathy and friendliness of staff.
- Team viability was the term used to denote the level of collaboration and co-operation between team members, plus the level of cohesion within the team.
- Task design related to the extent to which the strategy of care provided by the PHCT was based on the health needs of the practice population, informed team objectives and the mix of skills in the team, and was monitored and evaluated.

- Organisational efficiency was characterised by the extent to which teams achieved locally and nationally agreed targets within allocated budgets.

Within these areas there were 25 items relating to effectiveness. Respondents were first asked to rate each item in terms of its importance as a measure of effectiveness for PHCTs, on a scale ranging from 1 (not at all important) to 5 (extremely important). Secondly, they were asked to rate the extent to which the criteria had been implemented in their practice, on a scale ranging from 1 (not at all) to 5 (to a great extent). Box 11.1 below gives an example of the criteria used in the Primary Health Care Team Effectiveness Questionnaire (PHCTEQ).

Box 11.1

Some practices provide patient information leaflets setting out services available within the practice, information on how to contact a doctor or nurse during normal working hours and in an emergency. A few practices go so far as to provide patients with copies of the practice annual report.

How important is provision of patient information as a measure of effectiveness for primary health care teams?
To what extent does your practice provide patients with information?

The criteria generated constituted output (i.e. work activity) rather than true health outcomes (i.e. health gain for service users). Outcome measures proved to be beyond the scope of this research project.

An empirical model of primary health care team effectiveness

Figure 11.1 shows a diagrammatic representation of the empirical framework used in the research. Although health outcomes were beyond the scope of this research project, this aspect is included in the diagram for the sake of completeness.

The model is fundamentally causal and, although the direction of causality is indicated, it is acknowledged that the process of PHCT effectiveness is essentially a dynamic interaction between a vast array of factors. The framework suggests firstly that the structure of the PHCT in terms of the numbers of people in the team, the range of disciplines represented and the organisational structure (inputs) influences team member behaviour (process), and secondly that team processes influence team outputs.

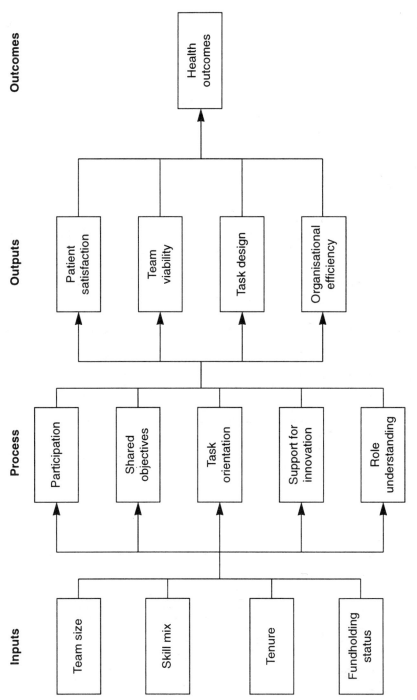

Figure 11.1 An empirical model of primary health care team effectiveness

Based on this empirical model, the aims of the research were as follows:

- to explore the relationship between team inputs (size, composition, tenure and organisational factors) and team processes (participation, shared objectives, support for innovation, task orientation and role understanding);
- to explore the relationship between team processes and team outputs (patient satisfaction, team viability, task design and organisational efficiency).

Method

An opportunistic sample of 80 PHCTs was accessed through the Health Education Authority Multidisciplinary Team Workshop Programme (Spratley, 1989) (see also Chapter 6). The final sample consisted of 720 members of 68 PHCTs in England. These included 66 district nurses, 140 general practitioners, 75 health visitors, 54 practice managers, 86 practice nurses, 168 receptionists and 131 others (e.g. midwives, counsellors, community psychiatric nurses, pharmacists, etc.) (Table 11.1). Table 11.2 shows the size and fundholding status of the participating practices.

The PHCTQ was sent to all members of the participating teams. Teams were only included in the sample if four members or 40 per cent of members

Table 11.1 Practitioner profile of participating teams

Code	Job title	Number of respondents	Percentage of sample
1	District nurse	66	9.2
2	General practitioner	140	19.4
3	Health visitor	75	10.4
4	Practice manager	54	7.5
5	Practice nurse	86	11.9
6	Receptionist	167	23.3
7	Other	131	18.3
Total		720	100

Table 11.2 Size and fundholding status of participating practices

Team size	NFH (%)	FH (%)	Total (%)
< 14 members	22 (32.4)	3 (4.4)	25 (36.8)
14–21 members	19 (27.9)	2 (2.9)	21 (30.9)
> 21 members	11 (16.2)	11 (16.2)	22 (32.3)
Total	52 (76.5)	16 (23.5)	68 (100)

FH = fundholding; NFH = non-fundholding.

of the team responded (whichever was the larger). The questionnaires were delivered by mail and prepaid return envelopes were enclosed. Six months after this survey, practice managers in the 68 responding teams were re-contacted and asked to arrange completion of the team effectiveness measure (PHCTEQ) by three key practitioners in the team (one GP, one nurse and one administrator).

Results

As discussed elsewhere, there was considerable variation in the size of PHCTs, ranging from the smallest, with seven members, up to the largest, with 37 members. The average size of PHCTs in the study was 18 members. However, there was a lack of agreement between respondents in several teams as to the number of people in their team (see also Chapter 10). In an effort to reconcile this anomaly, at the second administration of the question-naire we asked the practice manager or senior administrator to state the exact number of people in their 'PHCT'. We stressed that by PHCT we referred not only to practice-based staff but also to attached community staff who regularly attended team meetings and shared the same group of patients.

No relationship between team structure and team effectiveness was identified. There was a negative correlation between participation and team size. This finding demonstrated that interaction and participation in decision-making in the team was significantly related to the size of the team. In PHCTs with more than 14 members, the levels of interaction and co-operation decreased. Overall, team process factors were the most powerful predictors of effectiveness. However, more specifically, clarity of objectives was found to be the best predictor of PHCT effectiveness in terms of task design, team viability and organisational efficiency.

For a more detailed report of the statistical findings of this study, see Poulton and West (1996b).

Implications for the future of primary care

Overall, the research reported in this chapter presents a picture of the unco-ordinated approach to primary health care delivery that currently exists. This lack of co-ordination results in structures which do not facilitate a team approach. At the most fundamental level, most team members are not entirely clear as to who belongs to their team. Optimal levels of participation are achieved in teams with up to 14 members, yet most teams have more than 14 members, the average being 18 members in the sample surveyed (see also Chapter 3).

The model of PHCT effectiveness developed in this research follows an input–process–output configuration. The results showed a correlation between team size (input) and interaction and participation and decision-making (process), and between clear shared objectives (process) and outputs in the form of the structuring of PHCT activity (task design), how well the members worked as a team (team viability), and the efficiency of the team. In terms of these results, the model has proved to be a useful empirical framework to guide this research. Further testing with other teams has been undertaken subsequently, and is reported elsewhere (West *et al.*, 1994).

Although clear, shared objectives emerged as the most powerful predictor of PHCT effectiveness, it has been shown that current primary health care structures militate against the development of shared objectives. One problem concerns the multiple lines of accountability and management control in primary health care. Figure 11.2 shows a simplified example of current lines of accountability for members of PHCTs, and highlights some of the ways in which conflict of values and loyalties may occur.

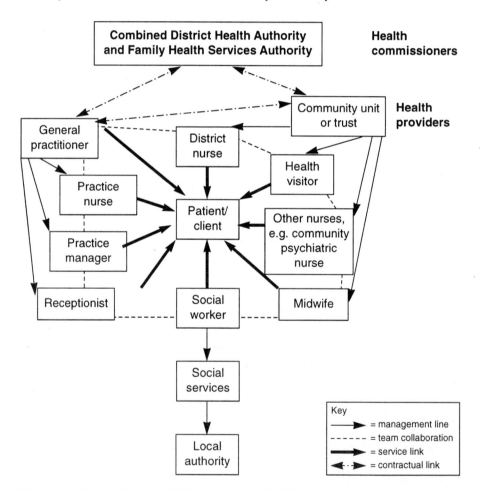

Figure 11.2 Lines of accountability for primary health care teams

For example, GPs – who are paid on a non-salaried contractual basis – inevitably have a different agenda in terms of objectives to other team members. This view is supported by content analysis of GP objectives, which suggests a bias in favour of maximising practice income, with services to patients coming a close second.

Practice-employed staff, although accountable to the GPs, have a link to Family Health Service Authorities (FHSAs) (part of the new Health Authorities from April 1996), which reimburse 70 per cent of their salaries. Therefore, even though practice nurses may broaden the scope of their practice, taking on more responsible roles, Health Authorities as controllers of the purse-strings are not obliged to reward this increased effort. Community nurses are managed quite separately by Community Units or Trusts. However, since the extension of the community and hospital services element of the GP fundholding scheme, some health visitors and district nurses may have dual reporting to GPs, who purchase all or a proportion of their services.

This unique structure makes it extremely difficult to achieve shared objectives within teams, because of the differing lines of management across the various professional groups. It would seem, therefore, that so long as the existing organisational and management systems persist, achievement of shared objectives and improved PHCT effectiveness represent an extremely difficult task.

A new model of primary health care

In the light of the findings of this research, a radical restructuring of primary health care is proposed, and this is presented in Figure 11.3.

Amalgamation of the community element of District Health Authorities (DHAs) and FHSAs has resulted in the creation of Primary Health Care Commissioning Bodies. These commissions would provide the interface between primary and secondary care, and set clinical guidelines which would inform the commissioning decisions of locality primary health care purchasing units.

Primary health care purchasers would be individual PHCTs which would have budgets devolved to the team according to the assessed needs of their practice population, based on a detailed health needs analysis. This model would differ from the fundholding scheme, as the budget would be controlled by the practice team rather than by a group of fundholding GPs. Within each primary health care team, a management board would be created, representing equally GPs, primary health care nurses, practice administrators (the term 'practice manager' should be avoided as inappropriate nomenclature), patient representatives and a non-executive chair drawn from the community. This management board would be responsible for maintaining a comprehensive practice health needs analysis, on which objectives for the team as a whole would be based. The board would also be

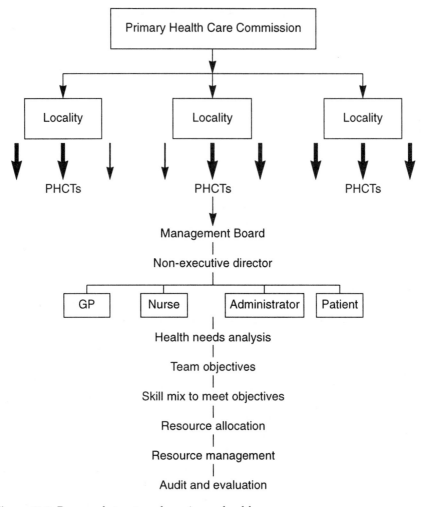

Figure 11.3 Proposed structure for primary health care

responsible for ensuring that feedback on the performance of the team was provided to its members.

In order to create equality, all team members, including GPs, would be salaried. However, it must be acknowledged that, as purchasing units, PHCTs are too small to stand alone. An interim locality tier is therefore proposed. A group of PHCTs would be incorporated into one locality. The responsibility of localities would be to produce locality profiles and to negotiate to purchase care on behalf of the teams in the locality.

Each locality would cover a population of approximately 50 000 and incorporate between 5 and 10 PHCTs. Some specialities, such as community psychiatric nursing and learning disabilities, would work across localities.

The bulk of administration in terms of salaries and travel claims would be handled at locality level. However, the flexibility should exist to allow teams to assume the level of responsibility that meets their individual needs and circumstances. Such flexibility should allow teams to devise their own skill mix, resource allocation and clinical supervision. The locality may or may not retain the training budget, depending on the needs and capabilities of the teams within the area.

The locality management team would consist of a representative from each of the PHCTs, together with local authority social services, public health and housing and patient representatives, plus a non-executive chair drawn from the community. It would also employ administrative staff, epidemiologists and professional advisers as required. With such a structure, national non-substantiated targets for health improvement would not be required. Targets would be agreed at locality level by practitioners and consumers, based on local health and social data.

The whole focus of this structure is on affording individual primary care teams the maximum autonomy, accountable primarily to their local population, but recognising their responsibility to manage their negotiated budget in the most cost-effective way. A range of substructures may arise within teams. For instance, client-based teams (e.g. for children or the elderly) may be managed by individual practitioners within the team, according to their level of expertise.

Conclusions

In this chapter we have offered an empirical framework for use by researchers and practitioners when assessing PHCT effectiveness, and we have described the measures used to operationalise the model. First, we looked at the assessment of team structures and processes using a Primary Health Care Team Questionnaire that included the Team Climate Inventory. Secondly, we reported on the use of the constituency approach to developing effectiveness measures for PHCTs. However, we acknowledge that these measures reflect outputs for teams (what they do) rather than outcomes (what they achieve in terms of health gain).

Our research demonstrated that smaller teams with fewer than 14 members interacted more frequently and participated more in team decision-making processes. The most significant finding of the study was that PHCTs lacked clear, shared objectives, and yet this factor of team climate was the largest single predictor of effectiveness for PHCTs. Our research shows that the current organisational structure of primary health care militates against a team approach, and for this reason we propose a radical new structure for primary health care. Such a structure will require flexibility of team roles, and will certainly challenge existing role boundaries. However, if we are to achieve a comprehensive primary health care service which reflects the

World Health Organization principles (World Health Organization, 1978) of equity, accessibility, community participation, intersectoral collaboration and cost-effectiveness, a radical restructuring of primary health care services is required.

Editors' summary

In this chapter, Poulton and West have examined questions about the effectiveness of primary health care teams, and have described a unique study which attempted to identify factors predicting effectiveness. They have developed and tested an empirical model of team effectiveness. Issues which arise from this are the problems that they encountered in identifying primary care team members, the significance of team size in fostering participation, and the importance of clear objectives in predicting effectiveness. The criteria for effectiveness used by Poulton and West are process-related, looking at output. Outcomes, such as health gain for service users, remain an area for investigation. Poulton and West make proposals for restructuring primary care services in order to integrate agendas. This fits neatly within the framework put forward in the primary care White Paper (Secretaries of State for Health, 1996) for pilot schemes, but will need careful evaluation to determine their effectiveness.

References

Anderson NR and West MA (1994) *The Team Climate Inventory: Manual and User's Guide*. ASE Press, Windsor.

Audit Commission (1992) *Homeward Bound: A New Course for Community Health.* HMSO, London.

Audit Commission (1993) *Practices Make Perfect: The Role of the Family Health Services Authority*. HMSO, London.

Bond J, Cartilidge AM, Gregson BA, Philips PR, Bolam F and Gill KM (1985) *A Study of Interprofessional Collaboration in Primary Health Care Organisations. Report No. 27, Vol. 2*. Health Care Research Unit, University of Newcastle upon Tyne, Newcastle upon Tyne.

Bryman A and Cramer D (1990) *Quantitative Data Analysis for Social Scientists*. Routledge, London.

Connally T, Conlan EJ and Deutsch SJ (1980) Organisational effectiveness: a multiple constituency approach. *Academy of Management Review* 5, 211–17.

Department of Health and Social Security (DHSS) (1981) *The Primary Health Care Team: Report of a Joint Working Group of the Standing Medical Advisory Committee and the Standing Nursing and Midwifery Advisory Committee (The Harding Report)*. DHSS, London.

Department of Health and Social Security (1986) *Neighbourhood Nursing – A Focus for Care (The Cumberlege Report)*. HMSO, London.

Department of Health and Social Security (1987) *Promoting Better Health.* HMSO, London.

Donabedian A (1966) Evaluating the quality of medical care. *Millbank Memorial Fund Quarterly* 44, 166–203.

Donabedian A (1980) The definition of quality: a conceptual exploration. In *Explorations in Quality Assessment and Monitoring. Vol. 1. The Definition of Quality and Approaches to its Assessment,* Health Administration Press, Ann Arbor.

Guzzo RA and Shea GP (1992) Group performance and intergroup relations in organisations. In Dunnette MD and Hough LM (eds) *Handbook of Industrial and Organisational Psychology. Vol. 3,* Consulting Psychologists Press, Palo Alto.

Hackman JR and Morris CG (1975) *Group Tasks, Group Interaction Process, and Group Performance Effectiveness; A Review and Proposed Integration.* In Berkowitz L (ed.) *Advances in Experimental Social Psychology* (Vol. 9), Academic Press, New York.

Health Departments of Great Britain (1989) *General Practice in the National Health Service: The 1990 Contract.* Department of Health, London.

Lightfoot J, Baldwin S and Wright K (1992) *Nursing by Numbers? Setting Staffing Levels for District Nursing and Health Visiting Services.* Social Policy Research Unit and Centre for Health Economics, University of York, York.

National Health Service Management Executive (1993) *Nursing in Primary Health Care – New World, New Opportunities.* National Health Service Management Executive, Leeds.

Poulton BC (1995) *Effective Multidisciplinary Teamwork in Primary Health Care.* Unpublished PhD Thesis, Institute of Work Psychology, University of Sheffield, Sheffield.

Poulton BC and West MA (1994) Primary health care team effectiveness: developing a constituency approach. *Health and Social Care in the Community* 2, 77–84.

Poulton BC and West MA (1996a) *Measuring Primary Health Care Team Effectiveness: A Pilot Study.* Institute of Work Psychology, University of Sheffield, Sheffield.

Poulton BC and West MA (1996b) *Team Process Measures Which Predict Primary Health Care Team Effectiveness.* Institute of Work Psychology, University of Sheffield, Sheffield.

Secretaries of State for Health (1996) *Choice and Opportunity. Primary Care: The Future.* HMSO, London.

Spratley J (1989) *Disease Prevention and Health Promotion in Primary Health Care: Team Workshops Organised by the Health Education Authority.* Health Education Authority, London.

Sundstrom E, De Meuse KP and Futrell D (1990) Work teams: application and effectiveness. *American Psychologist* 45, 120–33.

West MA, Poulton BC and Hardy G (1994) *New Models of Primary Care: The Northern and Yorkshire Region Micropurchasing Project.* National Health Service Executive Northern and Yorkshire, Harrogate.

World Health Organization (1978) *Primary Health Care: Report of the International Conference.* World Health Organization, Geneva.

12

Outcome measures for teamwork in primary care

Pauline Pearson and John Spencer

Introduction

Many of the chapters in this book, like much of what has been written about teamwork in primary care, assume that teamwork is, to borrow a phrase, 'a good thing'. They assume that primary health care teams are more effective than individuals or other groupings, and that their effectiveness can be demonstrated in improvements in the quality and extent of the care that they offer. West and Poulton have gone some way to question these assumptions in Chapter 2. In this chapter we shall take a more detailed look at what we and others anticipate the outcomes of effective teamwork to be, and discuss some of the problems and possibilities involved in measuring these outcomes.

Outcomes in the literature

Much of the earlier research on teamwork in primary health care is descriptive, providing little guidance on exploring outcomes. The classic study by Gilmore et al. (1974) provided a snapshot of the work of the nursing team in general practice at the transition to health authority management of community nursing services, but did not look in detail at outcomes. Bond et al. (1987) studied interprofessional collaboration in primary health care, but in practice examined the relationships of doctor–nurse dyads rather than the overall team. Again, outcomes were not addressed. More recently, Hutchinson and Gordon (1992) have described a study in Northumberland which used a postal questionnaire to investigate the views of staff in 20 practice teams about their context. Although the majority of respondents felt that they were part of a primary health care team, many indicated that their roles were misunderstood by other team members. The outcomes that the team might seek to achieve were not explored. In the USA, Wise *et al.* (1974) looked at the development of a team approach to family-centred health care in a health centre in the South Bronx. They suggested a self-renewing model of the health team. Effective teamwork, they suggested, would result in increased energy for patient care, and failures of teamwork would drain the team 'battery'. Whilst this is an interesting model, it is difficult to see how it might be operationalised.

The management literature provides some useful material on teamwork and team functioning, but says little about concrete outcomes. Belbin (1981) in his classic text examined the factors involved in the success or failure of created management teams. He developed eight 'useful types of contribution', and suggested that the roles required in any team would depend on the goal they were attempting to reach. However, the outcomes required of his teams were relatively clear-cut, and not easy to relate to the complexity of everyday practice.

Identifying outcome measures

Most of the rhetoric of government and professional organisations suggests that effective teamwork in primary care will make a difference to patient care, patient satisfaction and/or health outcomes. Patient care and patient satisfaction are frequently the subject of audit. Health outcomes can be measured in a variety of ways, ranging from extensive questionnaires to simpler scales (Wilkin *et al.*, 1992). Why look any further? First, because there are many potential outcome measures that reflect the diversity of perspectives represented within the primary care team, and some consensus is needed on the most useful ones. Secondly, because many of the available instruments require considerable resources to administer, and more pragmatic measures are needed. None the less, there will always be a trade-off between reliability (reproducibility), validity (does it measure what you want?), acceptability to all stakeholders, cost in time or money, and the impact on practice.

In late 1992, we undertook a study to determine some agreed indicators of effective teamwork in primary care. We decided to seek the views of an expert group, and used a two-stage Delphi questionnaire. The Delphi technique is a way of drawing out and sifting the views of a group of people who are experts in the key area of interest. The advantages of this technique are described by Linstone and Thuroff (1975) as enabling debate between individuals who have not previously been in contact, avoiding the outcome of the group being controlled by dominant personalities, and letting everyone have an equal say. In addition, we felt that it avoided placing too many restrictions on respondents and enabled them to define their own terms. Reid (1988) has described some of the disadvantages of the Delphi technique, chief among which is that, since it works by consensus, it is unlikely to advance 'cutting-edge' ideas, or those proposed by only a few proponents. The use of nominal groups, a similar technique of which we had some experience (Gallagher *et al.*, 1993), was rejected as a method because the costs involved in a national study would have been prohibitive, and tight control would have been required to ensure equity in debate.

A range of possible experts could have been used. For instance, we could have talked to policy-makers, service managers or teams reputed to be working well. Looking at the possible groups, we decided to access people involved in promoting teamwork in primary care. We made contact via Family Health Service Authorities (FHSAs) with the people that they nominated as the key individuals involved in teambuilding in their area. In this way we made contact with a wide group, including policy-makers, managers, practitioners and primary care facilitators. Each nominated individual was then asked to pass on two questionnaires to interested colleagues. This group, we reasoned, would be broader in its perspectives than any individual profession. It would consist of people who had thought about effective performance in primary care and would therefore be sufficiently committed to complete the two-stage questionnaire.

Figure 12.1 outlines the Delphi process. A total of 237 questionnaires were sent out to the 'expert' group, and 137 questionnaires were returned, giving a response rate of 58 per cent. The initial questionnaire asked respondents to offer up to five conclusions to the sentence 'a primary health care team is working well if ...', and a similar number of conclusions to the stem 'a primary health care team is not working well if ...'. The completed items were analysed by us using simple thematic analysis as described in Stacy and Pearson (1994), and a list of the top 20 key items was returned to each participant.

This time, respondents were asked to distribute 100 points between the items which they considered to be most important, in such a manner as to reflect the importance placed upon each individual item. Hence they could give each of the 20 items 5 points, rating all of them equally, or they could give all 100 points to one very significant item. In general, respondents put 10–20 points on each of 5 to 10 items. The list sent out in Stage 2 was presented in alphabetical order, rather than in order of apparent importance as on the first round. In addition to this numerical rating, each respondent was asked to suggest how the top three items on his or her list might be measured, and to identify some of the facilitating factors or areas of difficulty which might be encountered in making such assessments (see Box 12.1).

A further question asked about each respondent's current role and past experience of working in primary health care. A total of 80 questionnaires (64 per cent of the first round returns) were sent back.

Analysis of the second stage involved a simple calculation of the scores for each item, after which the suggestions for methods of measuring items

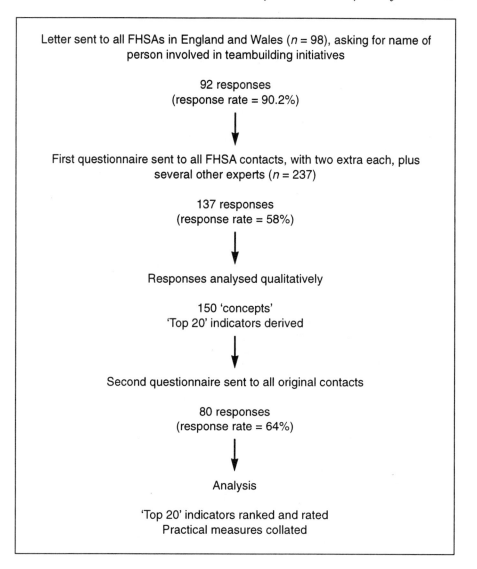

Letter sent to all FHSAs in England and Wales (*n* = 98), asking for name of person involved in teambuilding initiatives

92 responses
(response rate = 90.2%)

First questionnaire sent to all FHSA contacts, with two extra each, plus several other experts (*n* = 237)

137 responses
(response rate = 58%)

Responses analysed qualitatively

150 'concepts'
'Top 20' indicators derived

Second questionnaire sent to all original contacts

80 responses
(response rate = 64%)

Analysis

'Top 20' indicators ranked and rated
Practical measures collated

Figure 12.1

were listed and the factors that were considered likely to inhibit or facilitate progress were identified. Finally, the roles of each of the respondents were listed, and grouped, e.g. according to whether they were working in a primary health care team, a facilitation role or a management role. The results of this analysis have been published elsewhere (Pearson and Spencer, 1995). Table 12.1 shows the overall placing of key items. However, having completed this first analysis, there were two further groups of questions which seemed important to us. Many of those responding had stated that they had not worked in primary care 'on the ground'. We wondered

Box 12.1

In practical terms how would you go about measuring this indicator?

What problems do you think might arise?

What factors might facilitate measurement?

Are you aware of any existing tools which might help in measuring this indicator?

At what organisational level should this indicator be measured?

Table 12.1 Scores for indicators that a primary health care team is working well

Indicator	Summary score
A primary health care team is working well if ...	
There are agreed aims, goals and objectives	1272
There is effective communication	964
Patients are receiving the best possible care	682
Individual roles are defined and understood	629
There is appropriate use of skills	393
Members are involved in decision-making	391
There is mutual respect	385
Individual roles are valued	383
There are clear lines of communication	354
There is trust and confidence	289
The team is committed	286
Team members are involved in planning	271
There is open and honest discussion	262
There is joint audit and review	261
Regular meetings are held	257
Team morale is high	242
There is a co-ordinated approach	234
There is equality between team members	136
Support systems are in place	107
The team is innovative	87

whether managers and others without direct experience of practice prioritise different indicators of effectiveness to those who *have* worked in practice. In addition, although we had looked in broad terms at the suggestions made for measurement of different indicators, it seemed that a more detailed analysis should be made of what might be feasible in relation to key areas.

On the ground or off the wall?

Practitioners in primary care are frequently cynical about those in managerial or advisory positions. Was there in fact a difference in the views of the two
groups about a primary health care team that was working well? For example, did the group without experience hold more idealistic or unrealistic
views? What was the type of experience of those who had been in practice?
Table 12.2 shows the diversity of respondents who replied to the second stage
of the survey. Ranging from an FHSA administrative assistant to general

Table 12.2 Roles of the respondents to the
second questionnaire

Role	Number
Managers (FHSA/DHA)	22
Facilitators	21
Senior nurses	7
General practitioners	7
Health promotion staff	6
Practice nurses	1
Practice managers	2
Other/unclear/not stated	14
Total	80

practitioners, practice managers and a director of nursing, to a large number
of primary care facilitators, planning managers and project workers, current
job titles alone were not a sufficient indicator of where these people were coming from. However, the question which asked each respondent whether he or
she had ever worked in a primary health care team and, if so, in what capacity, was more helpful. In total, 52 of the respondents to this second stage (65
per cent of those replying) had worked, or were currently working, within a
primary health care team; 27 respondents (almost 34 per cent of those replying) had not done so, and one did not reply to this question. Of those who had
been or were working in primary care, one individual did not indicate in
what capacity he or she had worked. Table 12.3 shows a breakdown of the
remaining 51 respondents according to the capacity in which they practised.
The vast majority (83 per cent) had been nurses, and a perhaps surprising
number – 19 respondents (33 per cent) – had been health visitors.

What about the ranking of the 20 key areas? Was any difference discernible
between the two groups of respondents? We looked first at the number of
'votes' cast for any item, rather than the numerical weightings attached. In
terms of the areas that were voted for, 'agreed aims, goals and objectives' was
a clear leader, with only six respondents – equally divided between those
who had and had not worked in primary care – not giving this a vote.

Table 12.3 Roles of respondents who, at some time, have worked in a primary care team

Role	Number
Health visitor	19
GP	7
Practice nurse	6
District nurse	2
Community psychiatric nurse	2
Practice manager	2
Community midwife	1
Team leader	1
Primary care nurse	1
Health promotion nurse	1
Various roles (nursing)	9

'Equality between team members' and 'support systems in place' were the two areas with least votes, each receiving only 22 votes. In each case, fewer individuals with primary care experience scored the item, with 38 individuals leaving each area blank, compared to 19 people without field experience. However, this difference is not statistically significant. It appears to reflect the higher proportion of individuals with experience of working in primary care in the overall sample.

The overall ranking of the indicators by score (see Table 12.4) shows some areas of difference between the overall ranking and the rankings for the two groups of respondents, i.e. those with experience of primary care (Group 1) and those without such experience (Group 2). Whilst the two top items overall were the same for both categories of respondent, role definition seemed to be rather more important for the group with practice experience for than the others. 'Patients receiving best possible care' was valued highly by all groups, but slightly less so by those with practice experience. Valuing of individuals' roles was also seen as very important by Group 1. Trust and confidence in colleagues were also valued more by this group. Involvement in planning appeared to be rather less important for individuals who had been in practice. Joint audit and review, on the other hand, were perceived as more important by this group. Overall, the number of votes cast reflected the pattern of the scores, with all but six respondents (92.5 per cent) voting for aims/goals as an important indicator of an effective team whilst, at the other end of the scale, only 20 respondents (25 per cent) voted in favour of being innovative.

Measurement in practice

Almost all of the respondents to the second round of the Delphi survey completed the additional questions with regard to their own 'top three'

Table 12.4 Ranking of indicators by score

Indicator	+PHC experience	−PHC experience	Missing	Total
Agreed aims, goals and objectives	799	463	10	1272
Effective communication	623	331	10	764
Individual roles defined and understood	412	217		629
Patients receiving best possible care	366	296	20	692
Individual roles valued	266	127		393
Clear lines of communication	255	99		354
Mutual respect	254	131		385
Appropriate use of skills	243	150		393
Involvement in decision-making	241	150		391
Team committed	228	58		286
Trust and confidence	220	69		289
Joint audit and review	209	52		261
Regular meetings held	187	70		257
Open and honest discussion	181	81		262
Co-ordinated approach	150	84		234
Members involved in planning	149	122		271
High team morale	148	94		242
Equality between team members	105	31		136
Team is innovative	75	12		87
Support systems in place	74	33		107

PHC = primary health care.

items. Despite the attempt to separate out each of the items, three main approaches to measurement were commonly suggested. The most common proposal was some form of audit: setting a standard – e.g. for effective communication within a given team – and then seeking evidence that it had been met. Difficulties were envisaged with regard to obtaining evidence about issues such as verbal communication, or in gaining consensus between respondents about the level of fulfilment achieved. On the positive side, it was recognised that a considerable amount of work had already been done in the audit area (see Chapters 8 and 9). The second most frequently offered suggestion was that a questionnaire should be sent to all staff in the team, in order to determine the extent to which a particular item was being achieved. This is effectively the approach which has been adopted by Poulton and West (Chapter 11) and ourselves (Chapter 10) in the past. The difficulties envisaged by respondents were identification of a suitably valid and reliable tool, and achievement of an adequate level of participation. The third most frequently cited approach focused on the use of patient satisfaction as a measure. Despite our selection of individuals with an active interest or involvement in teambuilding and promoting teamwork in primary care, few of those responding to the Delphi survey could refer to any tried and tested ways of measuring the selected indicators.

Practical examples

In this section, we shall look at some of the ways in which it was suggested that individual indicators might be measured. Suggestions with regard to aims and goals focused first of all on written structures: 'all meetings to be minuted, therefore decisions, referrals, etc. would be recorded. All minutes could be reviewed and checked to see if action had been followed up' and 'written schedules'.

If aims and goals are not written down, it is more difficult to audit the extent to which they are being achieved. Written protocols may also facilitate communication. A further element was the importance of regular updating and review, which in the following example is linked to another area deemed to be vital – the ownership of aims and goals by all team members: 'A practice plan would exist in which there would be specific objectives agreed on an annual basis which would involve contributions from the whole team'.

This area is discussed in some detail in Chapter 7. A major barrier to success in this area was perceived to be lack of clarity. This included individuals assuming that they held goals in common, rather than being clear about their different perspectives (see Chapter 4). Another problem area was lack of a clearly identified responsibility within the team for carrying aims and goals forward operationally. If no one felt that achieving a particular task was their job, it would not be completed. Additional problem areas included exposing weaknesses to others in the group, and power relationships in the team.

Effective communication – a huge area – generated a considerable number of ideas about measurement. These included the use of specific means of recording messages, meetings, etc., such as: 'Circulating information and checking who had received and read it and knew the content'.

Regular meetings and updates were suggested, together with designated key individuals for information and progress reporting. 'Attendance at meetings' and 'return to manager of circulars by time stated' were among the ways in which effective communication might be measured. Ways of identifying weak points were suggested, e.g. delays in receiving discharge information. 'Patient satisfaction' was also suggested as a measure of success. It was thought that the Patient's Charter might in some ways act as a facilitating factor (see Chapter 7). A culture of regular feedback and meetings with clear agendas in which participants felt that they had a role was also seen as important. Problem areas included the difficulties of obtaining an accurate record of communication, and also the potential threat to some team members, particularly those with a central role in communication, such as practice managers, of examining its success.

Suggestions made for measurement of the achievement of 'individual roles defined and understood' centred on the importance of clear job descriptions – individuals first need to be clear about their own responsibilities, and then need a mechanism to share these:

Job descriptions exist for all staff. They are reviewed on an annual basis. There are agreed areas of responsibility. Meetings on a regular basis take place between the whole PCT to discuss a particular topic (e.g. management of a disease, area of health promotion) and each team member will outline the individual role and contribution to patient care/management that he/she can make.

Surveys or interviews of team members, in which they are asked to describe each other's roles and examine the congruence of replies, were suggested as a way of measuring success. Audits of internal referrals (e.g. whether they were appropriate and timely) and of 'gaps or overlaps' were also suggested. Problem areas related to definitions of the team itself (who might be in or out) (see Chapters 3 and 10), changes in role boundaries and the dangers of over-rigidity of role definitions.

Audit was central to many proposals for measuring whether patients were indeed receiving optimum care. It was suggested that audits of specific services might give some idea of the quality of, for example, asthma care. In addition, patient attendance at clinics, etc., completion of treatment courses and measurement of the quality of patients' health were suggested. It was also proposed that patients, users and carers might be asked for their views of the services offered. The problems in this area were the enormous range of potential outcomes, which require one to focus on more specific topics and themes, and also the difficulty of making a decision about precisely what was 'best care' – whether it should be defined from the viewpoint of a professional, a patient or a carer, or a combination of these.

Conclusions

The perceived importance of shared aims and goals and effective communication in ensuring effective teamwork is highlighted by this study. Furthermore, it is clear that individuals who have been actively involved in primary care teams are in agreement with those who have not that these two areas are of central importance. However, there is an element of disagreement about other areas. Why this should be is unclear. The importance of providing good quality patient care and of appropriate use of skills may, for example, be taken for granted by practitioners, and valued more by those whose interest in primary care is more theoretical or managerial, but there is no clear evidence for this. The importance placed by the practice experience group on roles being defined and understood may relate to their day-to-day experiences of uncertainty about roles within their own workplace. Within a context of changing boundaries, this is understandable.

Three types of approach to measuring effective teamwork have been proposed by the respondents to this study. Examination of written data sources – minutes, memos, etc. is frequently mentioned, perhaps because it does not involve additional data collection. Use of the audit cycle was the second most popular approach, with mention of agreeing upon, monitoring and reviewing objectives. Examining patient satisfaction was the third most popular approach, mentioned by many respondents. It will be important for researchers and practitioners to explore the practicality of each of these approaches further.

Most of the indicators in the list generated by this study remain indicators of process (what a successful team might look like) rather than of outcome (what they achieve). In Chapter 11, Poulton and West, seeking answers to a similar question, have highlighted how they ended up with a list of outputs (tasks) rather than outcomes. There remains therefore a significant challenge for researchers in primary care – to develop and test measures that genuinely identify the outcomes (achievements) of the groupings of people who work in primary care, and thus enable us to explore further the truth of the notion that teamwork in primary health care is a 'good thing'.

Editors' summary

In this chapter we have set out some of the findings of a Delphi study which sought to identify outcomes of effective teamwork in primary health care. We found that people who had experience of working in a primary health care team identified different priorities in ranking outcome indicators to those who had no such experience. Where civil servants and non-clinically based managers are charged with identifying effectiveness, these differences may be important. We outlined the three types of approach to measuring effective teamwork suggested by our respondents, and noted that further work is needed to explore the practicality of each of these. Finally, we pointed out that most of the indicators generated were indicators of effective teamwork *process* rather than effective teamwork *outcome*, and we highlighted the challenge still facing researchers in this area.

References

Belbin M (1981) *Management Teams – Why They Succeed or Fail*. Heinemann, London.

Bond J, Cartlidge A and Gregson B (1987) Interprofessional collaboration in primary health care. *Journal of the Royal College of General Practitioners* 37, 158–61.

Gallagher M, Hares T, Spencer JA, Bradshaw C and Webb I (1993) Nominal group technique. A new research tool for general practice? *Family Practice* 10, 76–81.

Gilmore G, Bruce N and Hunt M (1974) *The Work of the Nursing Team in General Practice*. Council for the Education and Training of Health Visitors, London.

Hutchinson A and Gordon S (1992) Primary care teamwork: making it a reality. *Journal of Interprofessional Care* 6, 31–42.

Linstone HA and Thuroff M (1975) *The Delphi Method: Techniques and Applications*. Addison Wesley, Reading, MA.

Pearson P and Spencer J (1995) Pointers to effective teamwork: exploring primary care. *Journal of Interprofessional Care* 9, 131–8.

Reid NG (1988) The Delphi technique: its contribution to the evaluation of professional practice. In Ellis R (ed.) *Professional Competence and Quality Assurance in the Caring Professions.* Chapman & Hall, New York.

Stacy R and Pearson P (1994) *Coding Qualitative Data: Validity Through Consistency.* Association of University Departments of General Practice Annual Scientific Meeting, King's College, London.

Wilkin D, Hallam L and Dogget M-A (1992) *Measures of Need and Outcome for Primary Health Care.* Oxford University Press, Oxford.

Wise H, Beckhard R, Rubin I and Kyte A (1974) *Making Health Teams Work.* Ballinger, Cambridge, MA.

13

The Liverpool intervention to promote teamwork in general practice: an action research approach

Paul Thomas and Lynne Graver

Introduction

This chapter describes an intervention in Liverpool which has been taking place since 1989. It aims to help general practice incorporate the principles of 'Health For All'. This entails changing the way in which people go about their work, so that teamwork and collaboration between disciplines are the norm, and equity and promotion of health would be as valued as highly as curative medicine. The chapter is divided into four sections, covering the underlying principles, the intervention, the reasons for the evaluation approach, and the evaluation framework.

The first section describes health as a holistic concept, and primary health care as a way of improving health that values collaboration between all involved. The second section describes the intervention. At the time of writing, multidisciplinary facilitation teams serve geographical areas to aid the development of individuals, services and organisations. They help health workers to explore their own work in the context of local health needs and local resources. Effort is put into teambuilding, model projects and multidisciplinary workshops. Motivation and acceptance of change are enhanced by appealing to the interests of those involved, and by repeated personal contact. The views of everyone in the target groups are continually amalgamated and fed back in order to form a shared agenda for action.

Primary health care development challenges policy-makers and grassroots workers alike to work together for the benefit of the system as a whole, and progress in this must be shown by any change intervention. The third section discusses some of the research difficulties that can arise during this process.

It argues that traditional science (positivism) alone does not have the power to evaluate this type of work, because of the number of variables involved and its evolving, creative nature. We suggest that action research has the potential required. A four-dimensional evaluation framework evolved from the most recent stage of the Liverpool project, which may be applicable to other situations. This is described in the fourth section, and is used to explore personal, service and organisational changes (both anticipated and un-expected) and their connections. We argue that a variety of methods must be used if an understanding of cultural change is to be achieved, and that they must be cross-referenced. These include the use of quantitative and quali-tative methods and consensus statements, in order to gain objective data as well as subjective and collective views. All must be viewed together to achieve a holistic view. All of the different stakeholder groups must have the opportunity to influence the choice of indices to be explored in order to gain widespread ownership of the evaluation, and feedback and review must be ongoing.

Underlying principles

Planning for the Liverpool intervention involved asking searching questions about its aims and methods, and in particular about the value of teamwork, the meaning of primary health care and the nature of development.

The word 'team' does not necessarily describe something beneficial – a team can overly protect its own interests and do damaging things to others, e.g. a team of thieves. It is only when the aims of primary health care are clearly stated that the point of teamwork becomes apparent. The inter-national conference at Alma-Ata in 1978 formulated the 'Health For All' principles, and these have been widely accepted as a cluster of mutually interdependent concepts. They include primary health care, health promo-tion, teamwork, equity, collaboration between sectors, community develop-ment and appropriate research and technology. The nature of primary health care can be inferred from this to be a means of improving the health of local people in a way that promotes equity and collaboration with the population. This inevitably involves teamwork at every level. The same Alma-Ata conference produced the now famous definition of health as 'a state of complete physical, mental and social well-being, and not merely the absence of disease or infirmity'. This reminds us that we all constantly draw on our personal mental integration, our physical capacity, our relationships and our 'connectedness' to act meaningfully in our daily lives. Primary health care must promote this holistic concept.

One implication of this is that primary health care cannot be a place or a group of professionals. It is a way of operating that potentially involves everyone – a way of thinking, or a paradigm, that recognises that health is everyone's concern (Macdonald, 1993). It is helpful to view primary health care development not as a set of bureacratic structures, but as a complex and dynamic system in which everyone values the contribution of others. A more limited aim (teamwork in general practice) may well help to deliver the medical and professional components of such collaboration (primary medical care) but, if developed in isolation, might also work *against* the more ambitious aim – developing the paradigm of primary health care throughout society.

If primary health care can be viewed as a complex, dynamic system, any intervention must acknowledge that it cannot reach all parts of that system – it is too large. Instead, it must focus on one part of the system and involve relevant, interconnected parts of this focus. An effective intervention will 'get the whole system in the room' (Axelrod, 1992) and thereby allow complementary changes in relationships and capacities within various parts of this focus. Inevitably, this involves the simultaneous development of people, services, organisations and their connections. Personal, service and organisational development are usually dealt with by different individuals because they involve different priorities and different methods. For example, organisational development involves teambuilding, and is concerned with people's roles, relationships and systems of communication. Personal development is primarily concerned with people's personal skills, including their confidence. Service development is not particularly concerned with people, but with measurable outcomes. However, everyone knows that in real life the situation is not so simple. Consider the example of immunisation – if the health visitor lacks the relevant skills, teamwork will not make the clinic run smoothly. Conversely, a very skilled health visitor is unlikely to increase the immunisation rates without practice co-operation and a regular clinic – these are all interconnected and interdependent, and they are all essential. An effective intervention to develop primary health care will ensure that people, organisations and services develop hand in hand – in this example to ensure that immunisation clinics operate regularly, with a skilled health visitor and with an agreed protocol which shows how each member of the team contributes to the immunisation effort.

This means that teamwork development in general practice cannot be seen in isolation from the development of individuals, services and systems. Similarly, evaluation must examine changes in each of these dimensions (personal, service, organisation and systems). Cultural change in this focal area can be considered to be the result of a new configuration of the system, in which people's behaviour and thinking patterns have shifted to gain a revised view of the world in which they live, and their part in it.

In summary, the Liverpool intervention aimed to change the culture of general practice towards the acceptance of the 'Health For All' principles (including teamwork) and the concept of primary health care as a complex and dynamic system. The purpose of these changes is to increase the capacity of individuals and organisations to address the health needs of local people; health is defined as an holistic ideal affecting all aspects of life, and of concern to all members of society. The expected outcomes of the work included improved personal, service and organisational capacities and their connections in areas of work considered by the various stakeholders to be valuable.

The Liverpool primary health care intervention

In 1989, as in most deprived cities, Liverpool general practice was for the most part isolated, crisis driven and disease focused. Despite some pockets of excellence, there was little teamwork and little in the way of co-ordinated relevant continuing education or support. The 110 practices (which included 240 GPs) employed only eight practice nurses in total. In addition, the health-involved organisations worked in relative isolation from each other – there was little history or experience of co-ordinated, collaborative work anywhere.

In an attempt to begin to address this situation, the Local Medical Committee and the Family Practitioner Committee (now the Health Authority) were successful in a bid for Inner City Partnership money to employ a GP and a nurse, with administration support, as facilitators for 2 years, starting in the summer of 1989, focused on the development of general practice. This project coincided with the start of the Liverpool Healthy City 2000 project, although this project was concerned more with community development and intersectoral collaboration. The two projects shared similar long-term aims and were useful to each other. By the end of Stage 1 (1991), a great deal had been achieved. For example, almost every practice had employed a practice nurse, a new practice nurse course had been developed, and six nurses were employed as practice nurse mentors. There were also many other developments, including health promotion initiatives, audit projects, and health needs assessment using a rapid appraisal method.

The success of Stage 1 of the project led to the start of the second stage, funded for 3 years, in the summer of 1991. A general practitioner, a practice manager, a practice nurse, a district nurse, an administrator and a health visitor, all employed on a part-time basis, formed the facilitation team and extended their target group beyond GPs and practice nurses to other disciplines. Conscious of the need to provide an environment in which individuals could achieve things for themselves, the team continued a 'bottom-up', problem-solving approach, by asking health care professionals and others what they perceived to be the major obstacles to progress. The information was amalgamated and fed back so that a consensus could be reached for action inside practices, across localities and inside the health-involved organisations. So, for example, practices and individuals with similar interests were put in contact with one another, and commonly perceived problems in practices were communicated to health service managers. In effect, the facilitators used a community development approach, in which the community to be developed was general practice.

This opportunistic, problem-solving approach continues to the present day, but the outcomes were difficult to predict, which made the facilitators and their managers feel uncomfortable. Moreover, it was not always easy to link the outcomes with the work of the Facilitation Project, since they were 'owned' by others who nevertheless felt empowered to act in a way that they might not have done if they had not been influenced by the project. With more experience and a greater understanding of facilitation principles, a number of packages of work were developed to make the effect of the work more visible. We have referred to these as 'process parcels', because they describe a repeatable process (e.g. residential teambuilding workshops) that would have valuable outcomes which could not necessarily be anticipated at the outset.

A 'process parcel' is a way of making a process appear to be an outcome. For example, a facilitated in-practice workshop, or 'roadshow', which explores any aspect of work the team wishes (say a diabetic clinic) is likely to have outcomes of benefit to the practice. It may clarify roles or solve prob-lems, it may identify new problems (e.g. the doubts staff have about its value), or it may galvanise the practice team to make changes. However, no one can be sure in advance what will emerge. It may be decided to close the clinic down! Outcomes can be described retrospectively, but this does not help to set targets for the specific outcomes of the work of the facilitation team.

However, it is possible to set targets for the number of roadshows to be held. Other process parcels devised included cross-practice workshops to explore problems and solutions around a commonly perceived problem (e.g. attachment of community trust staff to GPs), forums (cross-city workshops to explore the merit of a new idea, e.g. the employment of a complementary therapist), interactive bulletins (a bulletin sent to all members of the target group, with a questionnaire attached, the responses to which would be amalgamated and included in the next mailing), shared projects (collabora-tive and stand-alone projects in which various health workers work together on the same initiative) and repeated personal contact through named people for named practices. We also used the model of the residential teambuilding workshop from the Health Education Authority (see Chapter 6). All of these process parcels were multidisciplinary, and all of them could be (and were) counted.

A more detailed account of the work of the Primary Health Care Facilitation Project is contained in the report by Thomas (1994). Through repeated use of its models of operation, the Project was able to facilitate the production of diverse outcomes. The following examples may help to illustrate this.

- A practice roadshow explored what a practice achieved with regard to immunisation, and the practice identified that patients thought that the woman doctor was a man; this was subsequently clarified by putting the title Mrs after Dr.

- Most practices in the city took part in a workshop to enable them to write health promotion strategies, as teams, for the new regulations. This resulted in a relatively painless and high rate of uptake of the new banding opportunities.
- A forum identified that the major reason for the high cost of leg ulcer care in Liverpool was inadequate understanding of healing principles. This resulted in the development of a 2-year-long strategy designed to address this issue.
- Several practices (with a research worker) investigated attendance at Well Woman Clinics in deprived and relatively affluent areas, using an action research method. They found that they had an incorrect understanding of the reasons for non-attendance, and were able to re-focus their efforts (a shared project).
- A bus was used as a shared 'stop smoking' resource (under the management of the health promotion unit) with practices and community groups (a shared project).
- A total of 14 practices collaborated on a project in which patients were interviewed in the waiting-rooms of surgeries about the hazards they encounted at work and, as a result of the data collected, they developed city-wide campaigns for change involving trade unions, academics and politicians (a shared project).

These and other outcomes of the project were of value in their own right, but their most important effect was to help health workers to see how the contribution of others could enhance their own work. This resulted in an altered perception of the value of others, and a changed expectation about working with others. When a sufficient number of individuals have developed this way of thinking, the balance sways towards this being the norm – this represents a cultural change.

The success of Stage 2 of the Liverpool Primary Health Care Facilitation Project allowed sufficient confidence to develop for the initiation of the third and most ambitious stage, namely the Local Multidisciplinary Facilitation Teams (LMFTs). This started in 1993, as a 3-year project. Four teams each consisting of five members were employed from September 1993 on a part-time basis to help develop individuals, practice teams and services in geographical areas, making primary health care facilitation less of a project and more of a way of life.

Each team operates the five interventions or process parcels mentioned above, namely workshops, roadshows, forums, interactive bulletins, shared projects and personal contact, allowing the empowering, culture-changing work to be more readily visible (Thomas, 1993). In exactly the same way as in the previous stage, the outcomes have been locally relevant. For example, one of the teams identified a need for receptionist training and, through their organisational connections, has developed a relevant course. Another team assisted all of the practices in their area to develop an exercise prescription project in collaboration with a local sports centre.

All members of these teams are employed for 5 hours a week and work in the area that they serve. They attend a university-accredited course[13.1] and have an inter-sectoral 'enabling group' to improve the links with health-related organisations. One of the authors (Lynne Graver) joined as a dedicated research worker shortly after the beginning of this stage, and has worked with the diverse stakeholders to develop the framework for evaluation.

Reasons for the evaluation approach

An evaluation must be able to say something about cultural change. As described above, primary health care is not one discrete entity, but a complex and dynamic system in which everyone values the contribution of others and stops imagining themselves as being central to the total health care effort. Individuals begin to see themselves as part of a much larger alliance of forces, continually changing in relation to different issues at different times. This is a marked change from traditional ways of viewing health care, as a collection of separate disciplines or as a service with professionals at the centre. Evaluation needs to say something about this changing paradigm. However, it takes a long time to achieve cultural change, and evaluation needs to detect trends rather than aiming to discover a final Utopia.

So, for example, one of the aims of evaluation may be to say something about the extent to which policy-makers and grassroots workers collaborate for the sake of the system as a whole, or about the extent to which individuals gain a clearer view of their various roles in the whole system and about their relationships with others in these contexts. Evaluation may set out to explore the extent to which the contribution of others is valued.

Tangible service changes (e.g. improved immunisation rates) emerging from an intervention are of value in their own right, but evaluation needs to detect the extent to which they contribute to the achievement of the longer term aim, when visible service changes reflect an improved understanding of collaboration. So, for example, an improvement in immunisation rates that results from a temporary extra health visitor who works alone would not be significant in the long term. It can be seen that cultural change in this context means the same thing as sustainable development – the end of the intervention does not halt progress, because the capacity of the whole system is changed. When improved immunisation rates reflect improved use of skills as well as improved communication and team spirit, cultural change/ sustainable development has occurred. From the point of view of evaluation, measurement of this involves understanding the significance of the links between the personal, service and organisational changes.

Evaluation needs to be able to cope with the complexities of the intervention and its ambitious aims. The particular difficulty encountered by the Liverpool intervention is in involving and articulating the interests of the diverse stakeholders. The specific difficulty encountered when evaluating the intervention is how to get a handle on the multiple outcomes and comprehend their significance in producing cultural change. Both of these aspects have implications for the evaluation approach. These three issues need to be considered further.

Involving stakeholders

Evaluation is used to determine what happens as a result of an intervention, in this case the LMFT stage of the project outlined above. By identifying what is valuable, the participants and organisations can see and enjoy their successes, and by identifying what is not valuable, the participants can learn for the future. Both of these processes aid understanding of whether an intervention can be transferred to another place, and whether the intervention has been cost-effective. An important question to consider is to whom the intervention has been valuable. Developing primary health care means developing collaboration, which suggests that each of the stakeholders (i.e. those who have a 'stake' in the intervention) needs to find something that is valuable to him or her in the intervention. Therefore, all of the stakeholders must be involved in making judgements about the worth or merit of the work both at the beginning and as it progresses (Long and Wilkinson, 1984). The markers of change in which individual stakeholders are interested must be included in the evaluation, and each stakeholder must accept the chosen markers of others. They must also expect and value unexpected outcomes. This active involvement and follow-up means that the stakeholders become part of the research community. There are no limits with regard to what can be evaluated. However, effective and efficient evaluation must go directly to the heart of the matter – what matters to the various stakeholders. Effective articulation of the aims of the various stakeholders and monitoring of their achievements is important both for retaining involvement and for producing an effective evaluation.

Accepting multiple outcomes

Examination of the value of the development process from more than one perspective is not an optional extra, but essential to primary health care interventions, because different things matter to different people. The more diverse the stakeholders, the more the evaluation needs to recognise multiple outcomes – it needs to be holistic.

There are other reasons for desiring an holistic evaluation. Whatever an intervention may do to meet the aims of its diverse stakeholders, it must also aim to improve health. However, different stakeholders' understanding of health may vary. Evaluation can take account of this by viewing health in an holistic way, by providing an assessment of changes in health in terms of the mental, physical, social and spiritual health of the group for which changes are desired.

The context in which any development work takes place will influence the way in which both the development and its evaluation progress. So, for example, this project's effects cannot be understood without considering the Health Service reforms. An understanding of the context becomes another integral part of the evaluation. Evaluation needs to be able to say something about all of these areas (Graver, 1995).

The evaluation approach

Different objectives require different evaluation methods – something important may go completely undetected if an inappropriate method is used. A mixture of methods is necessary. Quantitative and qualitative methods with consensus statements each give different types of insight about the effect of an intervention, and could together provide a way of addressing the different priorities of the various stakeholders in the project. This has been called a portfolio approach (Beattie, 1991).

For example, policy-makers tend to view the system from the level of planning for services. At that level it is impossible to 'see' all the facets of the system, so policy-makers tend to value the use of figures as a method for measuring achievement across a large system. Objective quantitative measures are therefore an appropriate method for addressing their priorities. On the other hand, those involved in the system in a practical way are often more concerned with local issues in their immediate environment than with issues affecting the whole area. They tend to value how people feel, and the relationships between local individuals. Subjective qualitative measures are therefore an appropriate method for addressing *their* priorities. Cultural change in groups involves changed behaviour of the whole group, and not just of individuals. This is likely to be reflected in their communal statements. Collective 'consensus' views are therefore an appropriate method for articulating their shared priorities and conclusions.

However, the different sources of information still need to be pulled together to be able to say something about their collective effect. Review of the information by the stakeholders (or a sample of key informants) in general debate or in a specifically designed focused group can allow this to happen. An evaluation approach that allows the priorities of different stakeholders to be articulated and measured, and then used as the basis of discussion about the overall significance, could begin to draw all of the information together.

Traditional evaluation approaches have not had the power to consider change as a dynamic interaction between interdependent variables. Instead, change has been regarded as a string of fixed variables that can be measured and compared (Kingsley, 1985). This is because of the dominance of positivism, with its preoccupation with maintaining objectivity and control of variables. The problems related to the isolation and control of single variables also prevent the simultaneous promotion and evaluation of change. The participatory action research approach does not have these restrictions. In particular:

- it allows evaluation of complex dynamic systems with multiple agendas;
- it allows evaluation of unexpected outcomes resulting from the process;
- it promotes change through ownership and the use of timely feedback.

An action research approach was used to evaluate the Liverpool intervention because it was felt to have the power and the flexibility to enhance and evaluate change simultaneously in this complex intervention. In recent years, the predominant use of positivistic or conventional approaches to human sciences has been increasingly challenged. Action research and participatory methods have been advocated as an important approach to evaluation in health care (Baum, 1992; Poland, 1996). This is discussed further in Chapters 10 and 14.

In summary, evaluation of an intervention to develop primary health care is aided by a participatory action research approach. This must allow interaction between stakeholders (the research community) to shape it and to divine the cumulative effect of its diverse outcomes. It must take account of the local and historical context, changes in the physical, social, mental and spiritual health of the target group(s), and changes in the capacities of individuals, services, organisations and systems. The evaluation then becomes contextually specific, holistic and in synchrony with the needs of all of the stakeholders. The next section shows how the application of the participatory action research approach resulted in a programme of work and a framework for evaluation designed to meet the diverse needs of the research community involved.

The framework for evaluation

The Liverpool 'research community' is composed of a range of groups, including LMFTs, primary health care teams, voluntary and statutory agencies, and the funders of the development work and the evaluation. As the formal and informal networks of the LMFTs expand and the number of collaborative projects increases, more members become drawn into the community involved in the research, thereby expanding the system under study. In this way patient/client views are incorporated over a number of issues.

An evaluation constructed around the principles of action research has no set format. It can resemble many different things, because many different views have to be accommodated (Patton, 1981). It takes account of the context of the evaluation and it has a wide scope – it is multi-dimensional. A leading principle throughout the development and implementation of the evaluation framework involved maintaining the involvement and participation of the key stakeholders (Robson, 1993; Reason, 1994) through the use of facilitated work groups.

It was agreed with the Family Health Service Authorities (FHSAs) that a research steering group should be established. After considerable negotiation, this consisted of a small group of representatives with a commitment to feedback to other participants in the research community. The membership of this core group consisted of a managerial representative from the FHSA with responsibility for quality management, a representative from the Health Authority (from Public Health) with a responsibility for primary health care, two GP representatives from areas not covered by the LMFT project, two representatives from the LMFTs themselves, two members of the local Medical Audit Advisory Group, and the research team from Liverpool John Moores University (LJMU).

This group formed the key arena for dialogue during the development of the evaluation framework. In the initial phase their objectives were as follows:

- to determine what was understood to be the purpose of the LMFTs;
- to clarify the criteria for evaluation;
- to determine the scope of the research;
- to decide which were the most appropriate research methods to use.

An iterative process was developed whereby the local enabling group and the LMFTs were taken through the same process as the steering group. The information collected from these work groups was fed back to the steering group, who modified their decisions in the light of the additional material. In this way, the needs of all of the stakeholders involved in the development work were included in the creation of the evaluation framework.

The distinctions between evaluator and evaluated became blurred as the work progressed. Each stakeholder became both evaluator and evaluated. However, the evaluation required both co-ordination and guidance. One of the authors (Lynne Graver) was appointed as a dedicated researcher. The researcher's role was not that of an expert, but of a facilitator whose task was to support the development of each research participant's own knowledge and understanding (Smithies and Adams, 1993) as the framework for evaluation was developed and implemented.

The evaluation framework was designed to provide the most detailed picture possible of the development work. This was achieved by ensuring that it covered the areas of interest in a multi-dimensional (in this case a four-dimensional) way. It reflected the needs of *all* of the stakeholders involved in the development work. The stakeholders formulated the evaluation objectives in an overt and collaborative manner, and they participated in and received feedback during the evaluation process.

The framework was gradually drawn together by taking the material collected from each facilitated workshop and reworking it until a consensus was reached among the stakeholders. Four areas for consideration in the evaluation were identified (Figure 13.1). Each key area had a number of general objectives associated with it (the 11 boxes) which in turn contained more specific objectives. Inevitably, related factors started to appear in different boxes, reflecting the interrelatedness of factors in complex interventions. However, it was usually possible to distinguish the different elements to make the framework practical (examples of this are given in the text accompanying Figure 13.1).

As each criterion was identified, discussions took place on how the data might be collected and what would be an appropriate sampling frame (Graver, 1995). The choice of recruitment sample, the type of data collected and the methods used were therefore a product of the research process, and not under the direct control of the researcher. The framework took 8 months to complete, and remains subject to ongoing adaption during implementation, because development continues as the stakeholders clarify their needs as a result of the information fed back to them. Once agreed, the framework was taken forward for implementation and introduced to the teams recruited through participatory 'in-practice' forums.

Some outcomes could be anticipated, but many could not be specified at the beginning of the evaluation process, since they were a result of harnessing and promoting dynamism in the system. So, for example, the recognition that progress required general practice to see itself as a learning organisation evolved as the intervention developed. It is quite feasible to add this as a marker of progress, even though it was not included at the outset.

At the review stages, the research community has the responsibility to monitor progress in each of the defined objectives, and also to form a view of the collective significance of their simultaneous achievement. This is a way of reaching agreement about the extent of cultural change associated with the intervention.

Progress has been steady. Various participatory work groups became forums in which dialogue could produce consensus about the situation under study. Multiple evaluation methods were agreed, e.g. statistical analysis of the data submitted to the FHSA would be used alongside qualitative tools specifically developed and validated during the evaluation (these tools are authenticated according to the relevant research paradigm).

The following tools have been developed so far:

- the LMFT intervention records, which include facts and figures about the facilitation work;
- the researcher's PHCT check-list, which is a guide to collecting the background information;

1 Personal	2 Service	3 Organisation	4 The wider setting
(a) self-development, personal growth*	(a) improvement in the delivery of primary health care	(a) team development	(a) changing political climate
(b) the ability to facilitate	(b) meeting local health needs	(b) organisational development	(b) networking
(c) role clarification	(c) —	(c) effective collaboration, making connections*, working together*	(c) interventions

EXPLANATION

The framework which evolved allowed useful separation of component objectives in a complex intervention. For example, one of the priorities of the stakeholders is to examine what effect the project has on cytology screening levels. The framework allows the researcher to categorise the component objectives as follows:

- development of personal capacity to operate the cervical screening system (both clinical and administrative) in boxes 1a and 1c;
- the development of a robust recall system in box 3b;
- an assessment of the effect of the changing political climate in box 4a.

Another priority is to find examples of 'visible teamwork' within and across neighbourhoods. The framework allows the researcher to categorise the component objectives as follows:

- examples of shared activity or involvement in collaborative neighbourhood projects in box 3c;
- an insight into how clearly the primary health care team sees its role, in box 1c;
- an insight into how local health needs are being met in box 2b.

Figure 13.1 The framework for the evaluation of the LMFTs

- the semi-structured interview schedule, for interviewing the key informants in each PHCT;
- a statistical data trail for the PHCTs, designed to find specific data relating to health promotion banding and the levels of achievement of the cytology and immunisation targets.

These tools have all been piloted with one PHCT before being refined and used in the main body of research currently in progress. The programme of work for the evaluation to date is outlined in Figure 13.2, and further papers will document the progress of this strategy.

Conclusions

This research suggests that an effective evaluation of a complex intervention in primary health care should incorporate the following key principles:

- the employment of an action research approach;
- the use of participatory processes in the evaluation;
- the participation of diverse stakeholders;
- a multidimensional evaluation framework.

An action research approach using participatory processes seems to be an effective way of evaluating interventions in a complex system, because it enhances change and allows important outcomes that cannot be anticipated at the outset to emerge with the passing of time.

If the system of primary health care is defined too narrowly (and too few stakeholders are involved), any cultural change may only be relevant to a small part of the whole (e.g. to medical people), and therefore will not be sustained over time. This evaluation took a broader view of the system (involving more diverse stakeholders), which is resulting in a more holistic view of health and change across a wider field, incorporating new stakeholders as required by a specific phase.

Multiple stakeholders may become confused by the multiple agendas to be addressed. By using a framework that they have produced which incorporates all of the agendas, each is able to see how their agenda fits into the broader picture. This gives each stakeholder the comfort that he or she is being effectively considered, and also gives each an insight as to why other agendas are also important.

In this project, the research community found a framework of four different dimensions that were useful for encapsulating their collective views – personal, service and organisational dimensions, and the connections made with the wider setting (the context in which the evaluation is taking place). The framework helped to show how diverse outcomes affect cultural change.

Start of the evaluation February 1994	The key stakeholders were identified and the research steering group was formed.
Development of the framework February to October 1994	A series of monthly facilitated work groups was held to develop the evaluation framework. A key individual (Lynne Graver) was selected to co-ordinate the evaluation. The framework took 8 months to create.
Research methods March to September 1994	The evaluation objectives were matched with the most appropriate research method, e.g. service development uses statistical methods to identify changes in cytology rates, and organisation development looks at the 'systems' by using interviews, documentation, etc. The methods will be triangulated during the analysis.
Research sample September 1994 to August 1995	A target and comparison group of PHCTs and key informants was selected by using an adapted form of 'snowball' sampling (Sudman, 1976).
Research tools September 1994 to October 1994	The tools designed were as follows: • a PHCT semi-structured interview guide; • a researcher's general practice check-list; • an LMFT intervention record; • a PHCT statistical data trail.
Pilot study October 1994 to January 1995	The tools were tested and subsequently modified before use in the main research.
Developing the framework for analysis from the pilot data February 1995 to September 1995	This is a descriptive framework. It was the product of the themes that emerged from an inductive analysis of the pilot data.
The first report – evaluation of the LMFTs October 1994 to January 1995	A report designed as a device for discussion charted the development of the LMFTs and the process of the evaluation.

The first cycle of the main data collection March 1995 to October 1995	Quantitative data from PHCT statistics held by the FHSA. Qualitative data from LMFTs and PHCTs documents, interviews, etc. Consensus was reached during feedback activities.
Data feedback cycles July 1995 onward	The LMFTs, PHCTs and RSG all receive information and feedback from the analysis by utilising their regular multidisciplinary meetings.
Preliminary data analysis November 1995 onward	10 case records (4 LMFTs and 6 PHCTs) are being collated and then analysed using the descriptive analytical framework.
Evaluation continues to the end of the project (September 1996) and beyond February 1994 – February 1997	A second cycle of data collection and analysis is performed to establish what changes have taken place.

Figure 13.2 The programme of work for this evaluation

When primary health care is seen to be a complex dynamic system, both the intervention for change and the evaluation methods logically follow. A systems approach recognises that complex interactive processes develop a creative life of their own. Interventions that determine the outcomes at the outset can inhibit the desired creativity. A dynamic approach such as this one helps to soften traditional professional boundaries and allows roles to develop to meet the needs of the moment. The willingness to permit and welcome this marks professional cultural change towards collaboration and, as a consequence, towards the 'Health For All' principles. These and all other roles have the potential to change and to be shared. Here, for example, the evaluation becomes part of the intervention, and the intervention becomes part of the evaluation.

Editors' summary

The Liverpool intervention to promote teamwork in general practice was a relatively early attempt (taking place in 1989) to address some of the limitations of primary health care in that city by facilitating a more co-ordinated, collaborative approach to practice, and more consistent continuing education. It developed and expanded over a period of 5 years from two original workers to encompass four locality facilitation teams with 20 staff. In this chapter, Thomas and Graver have described the development of the intervention, and have detailed the evaluative framework that was used. They strongly advocate the use of a participatory action research approach to evaluate such a complex system since this, they argue, facilitates the development of a dynamic intervention which is responsive both to a range of stakeholders and to contextual change.

Endnote

13.1   The Certificate of Facilitation of Primary Health Care at the Centre for Health Studies, John Moores University, Liverpool.

References

Axelrod D (1992) Getting everyone involved. *Journal of Applied Behavioral Science* 28, 4.

Baum F (1992) Research for healthy cities: some experiences from down-under. In Leeuw E, O'Neill M, Gourmans M and de Brujin F (eds) *Healthy Cities Research Agenda. Proceedings of an Expert Panel*, pp. 18–25. RHC Monograph series No. 2. University of Limburg, Maastricht.

Beattie A (1991) The evaluation of community development initiatives in health promotion: a review of current strategies. In *Roots and Branches*, pp. 212–36. Paper from the Open University/Health Education Authority 1990 Winter School on Community Development and Health. The Open University, Milton Keynes.

Graver LD (1995) *Evaluation of the Local Multidisciplinary Facilitation Teams – The First Report*. Liverpool Family Health Services Authority, Liverpool.

Kingsley S (1985) Action research: method or ideology? In *Association of Researchers in Voluntary and Community Involvement*. Occasional Paper No. 8, pp. 1–36. Association of Researchers in Voluntary and Community Involvement, Essex.

Long RJ and Wilkinson WE (1984) A theoretical framework for occupational health program evaluation. *Occupational Health Nursing* May 1984, pp. 257–9.

Macdonald JJ (1993) *Primary Health Care*. Earthscan Publications Ltd, London.

Patton MQ (1981) *Creative Evaluation*. Sage Publications, London.

Poland B (1996) Frameworks for knowledge development and evaluation. In *Of and For Community Initiatives*. Centre for Health Promotion. University of Toronto, Toronto.

Reason P (1994) Three approaches to participative inquiry. In Denzin NK and Lincoln Y (eds) *Handbook of Qualitative Research*, pp. 324–39. Sage Publications. London.

Robson C (1993) *Real World Research – a Resource for Social Scientists and Practitioner Researchers*, pp. 170–86. Basil Blackwell, Oxford.

Smithies J and Adams L (1993) Walking the tightrope. Issues in evaluation and community participation for health for all. In Davies JK and Kelly MP(eds) *Healthy Cities; Research and Practice*. Routledge, London.

Sudman S (1976) *Applied Sampling*. Academic Press, London.

Thomas P (1993) *Liverpool Primary Health Care Facilitation Project; Local Multidisciplinary Facilitation Teams for Primary Health Care in Liverpool 1993–96 – Interventions.* Liverpool Family Health Services Authority, Liverpool.

Thomas P (1994) *The Liverpool Primary Health Care Facilitation Project 1989–1994.* Liverpool Family Health Services Authority, Liverpool.

Acknowledgements

We wish to thank Rose Sands and Conan Leavey for their helpful comments about this chapter.

14

Action research: a vehicle for change in general practice?

Harriet Hudson and Gaynor Bennett

Introduction

This chapter discusses two action research projects which focused on aspects of teamwork in primary care. The projects were conducted in Tayside during 1994 and 1995, and both were undertaken by Tayside Centre for General Practice, which is committed to a strategy of support and development for general medical practice and primary health care.

The first study sought to identify stresses experienced by members of a primary care team in order to facilitate more effective working. The second study was an evaluation of the introduction of a 'patient services manager' to a primary care team. It was funded by Tayside Health Board. In this chapter we shall argue that in an unsatisfactory world of short-term contracts and short-term money for add-on evaluative research, there is nevertheless an opportunity to pursue the important goal of using research to inform practice. The projects described below demonstrate the value and challenges of using an action research model, and raise a number of questions as to the future direction of such practice-based research models.

Qualitative research is particularly appropriate in general practice settings. The validity and reliability of medical knowledge have traditionally been rooted in a positivistic scientific tradition (Lowry, 1993). Medical education has aspired to confirm and uphold the importance of scientific rigour and certainty. At the same time, medical practice, particularly general medical practice as opposed to hospital specialism, continually grapples with the daily uncertainty of human existence, the reliance on the art of medicine as opposed to its science (Neighbour, 1992). The debate over the degree to which general practice is an art or a science has a long history and is currently reflected in the changes that are taking place in the medical curriculum at undergraduate level (General Medical Council, 1993). Many of the skills cultivated by general practitioners and by members of the primary health care network are those commonly associated with the expertise required of qualitative researchers, namely attentive listening, broad-based questioning, gathering information from a number of sources, formulating theories and testing them with a view to revision, and so on. Young doctors are taught to consult by history-taking, examination, diagnosis, information-giving and prescription of treatment (Fraser, 1993). These two processes are similar, and at our peril do we not make the parallels. These generally unacknowledged similarities facilitate the use of qualitative methods within general practice.

The experience of the two projects described here shows how easily action research can fit into the general practice field, despite being caught in the crossfire of a well-established debate about scientific validity and artistic licence. Whilst the debate will probably run and run, the practical outcome of useful and usable findings for practices to move onward and make changes is undeniable. In the end, action and outcome speak louder than words.

Denzin and Lincoln (1994) have made a strong case for the use of qualitative action research, both as an inevitable development of qualitative methods and as a practical movement towards local, useful research. They suggest that:

> The concept of the aloof researcher has been abandoned. More action, activist-oriented research is on the horizon, as are more social criticism and social critique. The search for grand narratives will be replaced by more local, small-scale theories fitted to specific problems and specific situations.

It is this approach that was taken by the two projects described below.

What is action research, or how long is a piece of string?

The traditional relationship of research to practice is that the research is conducted outside the arena of the practitioners. Practitioners then use research findings to inform their work at their discretion. Despite increasing awareness of the difficulties associated with this model (Reed and Procter, 1995), it is still seen as the 'gold standard' of research. In a medical context, gold standard research findings form the backbone of education and practice (National Health Service Executive, 1996).

The increasing preoccupation with dissemination of research findings is testament to a growing recognition that these findings are not widely adopted. The dissemination strategy has now become an accepted part of the research process, and is encouraged within research proposals. This is a welcome development. However, dissemination does not necessarily lead to implementation. The time scale of traditional research can sometimes discourage implementation of findings. There is often a gap between research field work, findings and dissemination that has an impact on implementation possibilities, encouraging the doubtful and discouraging the keen.

Research methods themselves can offer practitioners strategies for change and development. Research in this sense becomes part of a process of practice, integral to the day-to-day work of practitioners in the field. As the researcher becomes a practitioner – part of the group – research and development boundaries elide and overlap.

The medical research tradition suggests that research that is small-scale and interactive is not valid. However, action research in its widest sense may have something to offer to general medical practice, and may enhance the relationship between research and development.

Action research is a concept, and in practice can vary in different settings. Foote Whyte (1991) describes it well:

> In participatory action research, people in the organisation or community under study participate actively with the researcher throughout the research process from the initial design to the final presentation of results and discussion of their action implications. Action research thus contrasts sharply with the conventional model of pure research in which members of organisations and communities are treated as passive subjects, with some of them participating only to the extent of authorising the project, being its subjects and receiving the results. Action research is applied research. Some of the members of the organisations we study are actively engaged in the quest for information and ideas to guide their future actions.

Participative action research implies that the researchers agree with the participants as to what it is they are examining. It has a number of key elements that distinguish it from other kinds of research.

- It involves all participants in the research field.
- It is interactive.
- It consists of stages of research and action which are agreed or negotiated.
- It engages in continuous feedback and dialogue with the researcher.
- It sets out to effect change.

The two action research projects described in this chapter are informed by a number of methodological traditions. In these projects, action research was thought of as a concept rather than as a particular method of research. It has a flexibility which is extremely important in the world of general practice. It combines a number of features that give it status as a vehicle for change, within a setting in which change is an inevitability (and yet something that is resisted). These features will be discussed below.

Educational change and curriculum development

Action research models of evaluation have their historical roots in educational research. In this model, the practitioner (teacher) also undertakes the evaluation and development of his or her own curriculum. Since educational development requires change, a model of research and evaluation is required which allows for change and development within the framework of the research. The traditional model of research, in which the researcher stands outside the research field in an effort to produce an objective account of events, is not appropriate to the field of curriculum change (Stenhouse, 1975). Action research is increasingly seen as appropriate in other settings, such as community work and social work. The researcher–practitioner model of working developed initially from the notion of action research. The advantages of action research are that researcher and practitioners can develop a dialogue which helps to bring the intended change about as smoothly as possible and enables the change agents to use information from the research data to immediate effect. Action research assumes change and development.

Participant observation

Action research has been linked with a range of qualitative methods, particularly participant observation. Foote Whyte (1991) has developed an approach known as participatory action research, which combines the opportunities of participant observation with those of action research. He has used this approach particularly in community development projects in the Third World. The method has been used in a number of studies relating to the emergent doctor, and lends itself to complex organisational settings, such as medical schools.

Pluralistic evaluation

Smith and Cantley (1993) have illustrated very clearly the importance of identifying the different players in a given setting, who will all perceive the situation differently. The meaning of success can vary dramatically according to perspective. The pluralistic perspective enjoys enormous respect as a starting point for evaluative research. This approach, together with notions of change management and participation, has informed the action research projects discussed here. Both projects used observation and semi-structured interview as the central data collection techniques.

The country town practice

The impetus for asking a researcher into the country town practice came from a key practice 'champion' – one of the GPs – who had already identified a need to pay attention to the fact that all staff reported an increasing sense of overwork and stress. The researcher spent a day in the practice in order to reach agreement on the types of areas that could usefully be examined. These focused on the day-to-day life of the Health Centre. The aim was to identify the strains and stresses that were experienced by members of staff in an attempt to consider how workloads might be changed so as to reduce these tensions and thereby produce the most effective daily routine possible.

The research proposal was drawn up by the researcher, and it was agreed that it would operate in stages (see Figure 14.1). The participants were made fully aware of these stages.

Stage 1
Collect information about daily working patterns and find out how staff perceive their working lives. This is to be done by observation, and by discussion with staff, and would then be followed by a themed interview with each member of the practice team. This includes all of the doctors, the practice manager, the practice nurses and the receptionists (both part-time and full-time).

Stage 2
Invite the staff to comment on the interpretation of events offered by the research. Focus on one particular aspect of the findings that could be the subject of change and development.

Stage 3
Introduce a change or changes in working practice, and monitor its effect.

Stage 4
The researcher reports back to the staff on the effect of the specific change, and the group of staff collectively discuss any refinements required. The group can then focus on another aspect of development based on the original research, or choose to identify a different aspect. They can, of course, elect to do nothing at all. Eventually the researcher becomes surplus to requirements.

Figure 14.1 Research proposal – country town practice

Stage 1 – collecting data

Observation

During the first stage of the research it was important to establish a baseline. This involved developing a picture of the daily lives of all of the staff, what they did, how their roles interacted, and where the stress points occurred. This material was never destined for formal reporting, but helped to develop themes which allowed appropriate questions to be asked during the interviews. The researcher spent parts of some days walking around the public and reception areas of the Health Centre, making notes and asking questions. This allowed a picture to be built up of each staff member's day as well as the general climate of the Health Centre. Time was spent with the doctors, receptionists and practice nurses. The health visitors and district nurses were visited briefly, but as a result of various complications concerning access, which did not fall within the topic of this chapter, their role was not a focus of the research.

By spending time with different staff and in different parts of the research setting, it became possible to record differences in the pace and structure of the different staff days. The receptionists' day was task driven and resembled a spiral something akin to a corkscrew. The doctors' day resembled a Christmas tree, with a central trunk of patient/doctor consultation and a number of branches off that central trunk which varied in their density and complexity. The practice nurses' day fell somewhere in between these two images. The main difference between the work pattern of the doctors and that of the other staff was that the patient consultation took precedence over all other work and acted as a guide and, most importantly, as a safety zone for the doctors. When other demands and other work started to swamp them, they were able to refer back to their core work of consultation. The other staff were driven by endlessly competing demands, and had no area of their work which they could regard as core and central and upon which they were able to base their work structure.

Semi-structured interviews

From field notes of interviews, a number of themes or research questions were generated which formed the basis of the semi-structured interviews.

- How is the character of the practice perceived by individuals?
- How are the various jobs perceived, and are there common 'worst' and 'best' bits?
- What ideas do the staff have about changes?
- What prevents them from making those changes?
- What training needs do staff have, and how are these needs linked to previous issues?

The purpose of these interviews was to determine whether there were common meanings, difficulties or points of view that cut across the different roles, rather than to identify differences between roles. Common shared points of view could be used as the basis for change and development. All staff other than attached staff were interviewed, with the exception of the relief receptionist and the computer manager (this was for reasons of timing and mutual availability).

Informal discussion

Alongside the more formal methods for collecting information, there was a continuous informal discussion between the researcher and members of staff that occurred as particular questions or thoughts emerged. These conversations, which could be regarded as 'in passing' or corridor discussions, sometimes yielded the most interesting and spontaneous comments.

Developing analysis

Many of the difficulties concerning change that were expressed by members of staff at the Health Centre were associated either with not feeling in a position to make changes, or with feeling that suggesting or implementing changes implied criticism of colleagues, which was unacceptable in such a small and intimate organisation. These feelings are reproducible across thousands of small businesses, and were therefore entirely to be expected. The literature about teamwork is full of the difficulties of establishing a sense of team among people who have unequal access to power and authority. The additional complication of the power carried with the status of doctor makes it particularly difficult to instigate meaningful and consensual change.

Four main themes emerged from the qualitative research work.

- There was a need for protected time. This was expressed almost universally, although in different ways, and stems from a need to control uncertainty and the unexpected within the Health Centre day.
- Training and staff development was recognised by most members of staff as an important vehicle in working towards teamwork and decision-making. Whilst there were specific training needs, training was perceived as having a wider use in terms of staff cohesion and sense of purpose.
- All of the staff expressed a need for more information of one kind or another. It was felt that information would give authority to actions and allow staff to feel more in control.
- Finally, and crucially, there was an overwhelming sense that the patient was 'king'. Whatever the patient demanded should be aimed at and considered a reasonable primary goal for the Health Centre.

The country practice was the epitome of a practice caught in a tension between needing to respond on demand to patient requests and needing a structure to make daily working life more manageable, i.e. to limit the demands. At a superficial level, these two elements appear to be incompatible. Patients and their usually temporary world of ill health will, by definition, have urgent but changeable demands that are not particularly predictable or, indeed, definable. Primary health care organisations are thus in a continual state of change and development, driven by patients' demands as well as by Government edict. Although the voice of the consumer in health care can be a focus for alarm and tensions among service providers, it is also a force for change and creativity.

Stage 2

This stage involved collating and disseminating the ideas developed from the initial data collection. The staff were invited to a meeting at which they were given a short presentation and a report. Staff comments and feedback on the early analysis were collected during the meeting, and all staff were also given a copy of the report 1 week before the meeting. They were offered a list of possible actions to relieve work pressures. This list was started by the researcher and contributed to at the meeting. It was decided by the participants to develop a staff training programme and to opt for two of the 11 suggestions made.

Stage 3

This stage involved implementation of the agreed changes. The researcher's role here was to clarify the actions required of the staff and to continue to involve all of the staff in the changes. This is very much a supportive role, and switches the focus from the researcher as the instrument of change to the participants.

Changes were made to the front desk in terms of both physical layout and staffing patterns, and a new system of managing repeat prescriptions using an answerphone was introduced. The introduction of a staff development programme was put into practice, and an 'away-day' was also arranged, for which the researcher was asked to act as facilitator.

Stage 4

Once changes have been made, the researcher withdraws and allows these changes to progress. The researcher continues to keep in touch with the setting and, as agreed, monitors the changes. It is vitally important to give feedback and receive comments. Once the changes have been 'piloted' and monitored, further changes, or alterations to original ideas, may take place. This is all part of the work of the researcher, who continues to visit the practice and report back to staff on progress. The system whereby feedback and formal reporting take place is also a matter of discussion between the participants. For example, a short written report to the powerful players in the setting has a different emphasis and implication to a general workshop. Methods such as the use of video or audio cassettes for reporting and sheets for feedback are all possibilities. The relationship between the researcher and the setting is potentially self-limiting. As change takes place and systems are regarded as more compatible and acceptable, so the need for a researcher and more change diminishes.

In the country town project, the researcher moved from research to facilitation and back to research using methods of enquiry which are appropriate in a consulting room, a sociological study and a private sitting-room. The value of such movement to the measurement and analysis of a unique and discrete situation was evident. The action research not only highlighted dilemmas, but also facilitated change.

Patient services manager project

The second project, known as the patient services manager (PSM) project, highlights these features. In April 1994, a patient services manager was established in a Tayside surgery. The overall aim of the post was to promote the development of an integrated primary health care team which would enhance the effective and efficient deployment of practice staff, in conjunction with community staff and other providers, to meet the needs of the practice population. The main objectives of the post were clustered under the following four headings: teamwork and collaboration, needs assessment, service development and team management. There were specific objectives under each of these headings (see Figure 14.2). An evaluation of this initiative, funded by Tayside Health Board, aimed to describe the strategies adopted and progress made towards the PSM's key objectives over the year's post.

Teamwork and collaboration

- To develop an integrated primary health care team through communication and teamwork.
- To improve communication between the primary care team and other agencies, including the social work department and mental health team.

Needs assessment

- To develop a practice population needs assessment to facilitate service advancement.

Service development

- To develop health promotion and chronic disease management in the practice.
- To expand the range and accessibility of services for all practice patients.

Team management

- To develop a management structure for all practice-based nurses.
- To establish an education, research and training resource within the practice.
- To expand the role of contract monitoring.

Figure 14.2 Patient services manager – objectives

Methods

The PSM initiative as framed did not lend itself to a traditional evaluative method. The general objectives of the initiative were broad, and needed to be operationalised once the PSM was in post. It was unlikely that all of the objectives would proceed at the same pace or be given equal priority by the PSM and the practice. The evaluative method adopted therefore needed to be flexible. An action research paradigm was identified as the most appropriate for the purpose. A number of methods, which come under the broad umbrella of 'action research', were used to describe the development of the PSM's role.

Regular contact with the PSM

The researcher made monthly 1-day visits to the practice. Each visit involved discussion with the PSM of key events (progress or setbacks) that had taken place during the previous month. An agenda was developed to ensure that all areas of development were covered on each occasion.

Document analysis

At each monthly meeting, documentation (e.g. meeting minutes, hand-outs and correspondence) relating to each of the issues discussed with the PSM was collected and subsequently used to illuminate key events further.

Interviews

The primary care team's perceptions of the PSM's role, as well as their attitudes towards each of his key objectives, were explored by semi-structured interview. Interviews were conducted with the practice manager, practice nurses, GP, health visitors and district nurses.

Observation

Where possible, formal and informal meetings and discussions were attended by the researcher.

Workshops and reports

In conjunction with the delivery of an interim report, the researcher held a workshop at the surgery at which thoughts and issues surrounding the PSM's progress and developing role were discussed. The workshop setting allowed the researcher, PSM and primary care team to discuss more widely the changes taking place in practice organisation, and to ensure that the research was addressing key issues. The practice was also offered the opportunity to discuss the conclusions and recommendations of the final report in a workshop setting.

The PSM's key activities

Both the interim and final reports described the PSM's key activities in relation to each of his main objectives, followed by a discussion of themes and issues arising from his work within the practice. On the basis of these themes and issues, interim and final conclusions were drawn. The relationship between the researcher and the key players was fundamental, as the researcher became a facilitator for the entire project, including the patient services manager.

One of the PSM's first priorities was to attempt to improve communication and teamwork within the practice. He believed that improved systems of internal communication would facilitate work towards other objectives. Meetings represented one of the main tools utilised to encourage increased communication. The PSM not only introduced new meetings involving the practice nurses and community nurses, but also attempted to expand the scope of some existing regular meetings within the practice. He experienced difficulties in trying to establish dialogue between the GPs and the community nurses within existing structures. The main recommendation of the interim report was that a strategic planning meeting should be established at which multidisciplinary discussion of practice issues could take place. This recommendation was responded to by the practice, and the first strategic planning meeting was held 2 months later. The aim of the meeting was as follows:

> To involve all the primary health care team in developing an integrated approach to the care of patients, to formulate and implement future plans and to give everyone a stake in that future. It is hoped that the Strategic Planning Meetings will provide a forum for discussion which will lead to teambuilding and teamwork as smaller, more functional, task-oriented groups are formed to tackle issues arising.

The first strategic planning meeting was held in the evening after surgery hours in order to ensure that it could be given the undivided attention of those attending, and to maximise the opportunity for all to take part. Reception staff, district nurses, health visitors, practice nurses, the practice manager, PSM and GPs turned out in force, and the researcher attended as an observer. The meeting commenced with the PSM giving a general introduction to the overall aim of the strategic planning meetings. He expressed the hope that it would give everyone a broad view of the philosophy and aims of the practice, and that this would ultimately lead to everyone pulling in the same direction. It was also hoped that improved communication would break down barriers and eventually result in better teamwork.

Four short presentations were made by the GPs. The first of these outlined the philosophy of the practice. It was emphasised that the practice was a business and, as such, its ultimate aim was to maximise profit. The second presentation continued the business theme, but distinguished between profit for the benefit of the GPs and profit for the benefit of the practice, i.e. it was pointed out that a large proportion of the profit made by the practice was ploughed back into service provision for the benefit of the patients. The third presentation highlighted obligations placed on the practice by the GP Contract. In particular, health promotion activities were identified as a strategic area of development for the future. The fourth and final presentation highlighted the potential role of the community nurses in assisting the practice to improve cost and efficiency of prescribing within the practice. The importance of collaboration with, and the co-operation of, the community nurses in helping the practice to streamline costs in the use of wound management products, immunological products, dressings, incontinence appliances, etc., was highlighted.

There was a very positive reaction to the first strategic planning meeting. All of the staff found the presentations by the GPs useful and interesting. Many indicated that it had been a useful orientation with regard to the needs of the practice as a whole. The atmosphere was constructive, and genuine enthusiasm for moving forward in a collaborative way appeared to be engendered.

A second meeting was held four months later. Again, the rate of attendance of practice staff was excellent, although a number of district nurses did not or were unable to attend. Four main issues were discussed: the now completed practice profile, health promotion targets, tetanus vaccinations and new premises. The health visitors outlined the scope of the recently completed practice profile, and they emphasised the value of the profile as an aid to planning future services. They also highlighted the need for the wider involvement of other practice staff in expanding and updating the profile.

The two strategic planning meetings held during the period of the evaluation were well attended and generated lively discussion within the practice on a number of issues. Most of those who attended the meetings stated that they were interesting, informative, and an economical way of keeping in touch with practice developments. On the negative side, some of the community nurses stated that they had not found the meeting a conducive environment in which to discuss controversial issues concerning their position within the practice, due to the presence of the practice nurses and reception staff. However, this probably missed the point of the strategic planning meeting. It seemed best used as a means of highlighting issues that required further discussion. Arrangements could then have been made for the community nurses and GPs to meet subsequently, in order to discuss these issues without the reception staff and practice nurses being present.

During the period of the research, the strategic planning meetings did not create 'smaller, more functional, task-oriented groups to tackle issues arising'. This was partly a function of reluctance on the part of those attending to volunteer for tasks when invited to do so, but was also possibly due to the fact that the tasks for which they were asked to volunteer (e.g. to maintain and expand the practice profile) were too open-ended. Many of the presentations made at the meetings highlighted the need for action to be taken, but without suggesting a specific plan. The final report suggested that it was the responsibility of those highlighting a need for service developments to propose a plan which could be debated within the meeting. Action plans developed through this debate could then be divided into task elements and formally agreed. It would then be the responsibility of those with the appropriate skills to come forward and take on responsibility for specific elements of the plan. It was concluded that a more structured approach to problem-solving within the meeting – one which created discrete task elements of manageable size – would help to overcome reluctance on the part of staff to come forward and volunteer. It was further suggested that, if the strategic planning meeting was to become a successful planning initiative within the practice, it was essential that it was not viewed as an end in itself, but rather as a means to an end. The planning meetings should spawn further meetings and should generate specific actions with deadlines, with named individuals assigned the responsibility of achieving them. Without a more task-oriented approach, the meetings could degenerate into a talking shop, and nothing would be achieved.

Unfortunately, the end of the evaluation coincided with the departure of the PSM to a new post. The extent to which the recommendations of the final report were implemented by the practice in the absence of a PSM to take the initiative forward remains unclear.

Discussion

The generators of both projects described above were GPs who were reacting to immediate work pressures and the short-term availability of money to support innovative 'change' projects in practice. The ideas behind the projects were rooted in crisis management. Both were highly ambitious yet unsophisticated ideas. They lacked understanding of the breadth and complexity of health centre life, and of the difficulties encountered in bringing about change and teamwork, which are well documented in the research literature (see, for example, Chapter 2). Workers involved in day-to-day practice rarely have the time or the inclination to take a step back from the coalface to view the broader picture. The PSM concept outlined in the early job description was far too ambitious, and lacked any direction or insight as to how the objectives could be achieved over a short period of 1 year. Consultation with a researcher/facilitator at the stage of developing the ideas for the project could have produced a more manageable project.

The advantage of early involvement of a researcher is demonstrated in part in the country town study where the researcher was invited in prior to any fixed ideas being set. In this case, the researcher was able to get a feel for the issues and to involve staff generally in identifying the core of the problem. The researcher was also able to mediate between the enthusiasm of one participant and the timidity of others. In Health Centre settings, the doctors are viewed as powerful figures whether or not they welcome that label. A researcher can act as a balance to the inevitable unequal access to knowledge and status that sometimes results in the bypassing of good ideas produced by participants who have little power. Equally, there is a danger that ideas promoted with enthusiasm by powerful players will be seen as the only options in a given situation.

The PSM project outline had already been decided by one person, who was a doctor. This did not facilitate a project that was essentially concentrating on teambuilding! The enormity of the issues under consideration should not be underestimated. The issues which the PSM was expected to tackle, particularly those of teamwork, collaboration and team management, have created difficulties within general practice for decades. The objectives of the project should have been tailored to the time period allotted, or vice versa. If the objectives are broadly based and ambitious, then a longer time period should be allowed for them to be achieved, with a staged action plan established by the 'interested' parties which is itself capable of change and development. Facilitative action research allows for a redefining and refinement of tasks based on participants' perspectives at any stage of the project. Consequently, the PSM project was able to utilise action research, despite the PSM project's rigid and unilateral set-up. In the case of the country town practice, the objectives were negotiated with all members of the health centre as part of the research procedure. This meant that in both cases, to different degrees, the facilitative/research role shaped and influenced the process and outcome of teamwork. Research-based facilitation was part of the mechanism of teamwork, not just an account of it. This is consistent with qualitative methods of research in which researchers become part of the setting, as well as observing it.

The nature of qualitative methods is such that their use seems to attract those who are able to live with uncertainty, and who have an interest in the underlying meaning of specific situations. Accounts of the development of qualitative research methods indicate that the 'search for the other' is also a 'search for self' (Denzin and Lincoln, 1994). This suggests that the types of individuals who are successful in qualitative research situations will probably also be successful in facilitative situations where the skills required are similar. Crucial to the success of both qualitative research processes and facilitative processes is instilling trust and confidence in the people involved.

There were a number of challenges specific to these research projects which are familiar to all qualitative researchers. In particular, there are issues of confidentiality concerned with achieving a balance between on- and off-the-record discussion. Clarity about the role of the researcher is essential for developing the appropriate balance here. The process of leaving the research setting was organised differently for the two projects. In the PSM project, the study period came to an end with the funding, and the PSM departed to a new post. In the country town study, facilitation continues informally. The relationship between the researcher and the practice has extended to being able to ask the practice to help in other ways related to primary health care, e.g. allowing teaching to take place in the health centre. The practice has become a fertile territory for development of a whole range of ideas. Whilst the whole point of action research is that it provides the best possible chance of putting research into practice, it still requires energy and commitment from all participants. Testing new strategies and holding one's nerve in tense and stressful day-to-day health centre life requires a 'product champion'. This can be seen as a useful role for the researcher/facilitator. The monitoring of changes is also part of the research. In the PSM project the changes stopped with the departure of the PSM, whereas in the country town study the changes stop when the facilitator stops asking questions.

Finally, it is worth reiterating some of the advantages of action research. The action researcher can be involved at the very beginning of the research and engage in the involvement of participants in change. He or she can arrive at any stage of the research and still be involved in its progress. Action research has a natural sympathy with general practice once the initial barriers have been removed. It delivers research findings and transforms them into practice. The degree to which action research becomes facilitation is dependent on each particular setting. In any case, those undertaking action research need specific skills, namely an ability to observe, record, provide feedback, listen attentively, devise open-ended questions, ask searching questions in such a way as not to alienate the participants, and develop trust within the setting which will not be abused, but used to develop the changes required. These skills are not easily acquired and need constant attention, but the pay-off may be a research method that can respond to practice need.

Editors' summary

In this chapter, Hudson and Bennett have set out the details of two practice-based projects designed to examine aspects of promoting team effectiveness, and they have explored some of the pros and cons of looking at innovation and change using a participatory action research approach. In particular, they highlight the difficulties presented by the crisis-based and unsophisticated origins of the projects, the need to involve an evaluator earlier in the development of any new project, and the evaluator's potential role in acting as a balance for unequally distributed power in a group or team – although this may mean developing a more distant relationship with the study's commissioners. Finally, they highlight some of the skills required by those utilising action research, and they suggest that where these skills are well used, this approach will respond to practice need.

References

Denzin N and Lincoln Y (1994) *Handbook of Qualitative Research*. Sage, Thousand Oaks, CA.

Foote Whyte W (1991) *Participatory Action Research*. Sage, Beverly Hills, CA.

Fraser R (ed.) (1993) *Clinical Method: a General Practice Approach*, 2nd edn. Butterworth-Heinemann, Oxford.

General Medical Council (1993) *Recommendations On Change In Undergraduate Medical Education*. General Medical Council, London.

Lowry S (1993) *Medical Education*. BMJ Publishing, London.

National Health Service Executive (1996) *Promoting Clinical Effectiveness*. National Health Service Executive, London.

Neighbour R (1992) *Inner Apprentice*. Kluwer, Boston, MA.

Reed J and Procter S (eds) (1995) *Practitioner Research in Health Care*. Chapman & Hall, London.

Smith G and Cantley C (1993) Pluralistic evaluation: a study in day care for the elderly mentally infirm. In *Research Highlights*. Aberdeen University, Aberdeen.

Stenhouse L (1975) *An Introduction to Curriculum Research and Development*. Heinemann, London.

15

Primary health care – visions and agendas . . .

Pauline Pearson

Development and change

During the genesis of this book, a great deal of development has occurred in primary and community care. The impact of a range of policy shifts has begun to make itself felt in practice. Further change is envisaged as I write, with the White Paper entitled *Choice and Opportunity – Primary Care: The Future* (National Health Service Executive, 1996a). Some of the key areas of change in recent years were outlined in Chapter 1. In this chapter I shall discuss the implications of those changes for teamwork in primary health care, and offer a vision of primary health care in the millennium and beyond. Finally, I shall seek to present the research agendas which this vision generates.

The 1996 discussion paper, *Primary Care: The Future* (National Health Service Executive, 1996b), highlighted the key philosophies underpinning primary health care. Drawing on the 1978 Alma-Ata agreement (World Health Organization, 1978), it suggested that primary health care should be seen as broad-based and collaborative, involving a variety of agencies, as well as being participative, engaging patients in planning and evaluating their own care. Multidisciplinary working was mentioned in relation both to the negotiation of changing role boundaries and to the need – as primary care team membership expands to meet the demands placed upon it – to educate practitioners from a variety of disciplines to work together effectively. However, the notion of teamwork requires exploration in many more areas.

The establishment of a central research and development function for the NHS followed a period of concern that much practice was not clearly research-based. A variety of reasons had been advanced for this, including lack of appropriately focused research, lack of effective communication by researchers, and lack of sufficiently substantial work in many areas. Nowhere was this more apparent than in primary and community care – long the Cinderella of health services research. Alongside the subsequent growth of NHS research and development, recent years have therefore seen increasing attention being focused on the development of research-based guidelines in primary care (Grimshaw and Russell, 1993) and, latterly, on the development of evidence-based practice in primary care (Jones *et al.*, 1996). Primary care practitioners are being encouraged to develop their skills in critically appraising research, and are more frequently questioning the assumptions that they have held for years. There is therefore an increasing demand for evidence about organisational structures, processes and outcomes, and about practice itself – does teamwork really make a difference to patients?

A further question which has begun to surface in recent years, since the Griffiths Report (Department of Health and Social Services, 1983), concerns how the patient, and indeed the carer, fit into and interface with the primary health care team. Early initiatives on patient participation in general practice appear to have been most successful in middle-class areas with articulate consumers (Pietroni and Chase, 1993). Community development approaches, on the other hand, have enabled such diverse groups as health visitors, midwives, social workers and dietitians to work with more economically disadvantaged groups, integrating their concerns and priorities into the process of agenda setting for health care in the community (Evans, 1987; Boyd *et al.*, 1993). The growth of locality purchasing (see Chapter 1) seems likely to gain by using this approach in order to produce genuinely participative decisions about needs and priorities. The community development model moves beyond the traditional primary health care team, and links agencies and local people together into a wider primary care matrix, presenting different challenges for research. The McMaster University System-Linked Research Programme and the King's Fund Whole Systems Initiative are two well-known attempts to address these challenges constructively.

The key players in the White Paper, *Choice and Opportunity – Primary Care: The Future* (National Health Service Executive, 1996a) remain more traditionally based around general practice. However, patients and their effective care are seen as central to development, alongside health professionals and managers. Although this White Paper is heavily focused on GP contracting, it clearly also assumes that a 'team-based approach . . . is essential to good quality primary care'. It advocates the development of a range of pilot schemes to explore alternative models of organisation and contracting, and envisages that many of these will incorporate nurses, midwives, health visitors and professions allied to medicine. Among the possibilities discussed for such pilot schemes are salaried GPs, practice-based contracts (implicitly permitting GP–nurse partnerships) and new roles for community pharmacists. Alongside this lies an awareness of the increasing use of private finance initiatives to develop NHS buildings and services. A further White

Paper is intended to take forward broader proposals in relation to matters discussed in *Primary Care: The Future*.

One new role which has been very much at the forefront in recent years is that of the nurse practitioner in primary care. This, too, may be advanced through the flexibility advocated in the White Paper. However, there is still considerable confusion about the role in the UK. Since Stilwell's original work (1982), her ideas have been hijacked by a number of different players. Financial constraints and, in particular, the reduction in junior doctors' hours have led to a mushrooming of 'nurse practitioners' in secondary care, not only in accident and emergency, but also in areas such as urology, paediatrics and ophthalmology. In many such expansions the nursing base for the post is unclear, in some cases leading to the undesirable situation where there are no nurses at all to provide advice or support. Although this has been less common in primary care, professional accountability and frameworks for decision-making remain important issues for clarification.

Meanwhile, practice nurses' numbers have increased many times (Ross *et al.*, 1994) since the advent of the 1990 GP Contract (Department of Health and the Welsh Office, 1989). Some feel ill prepared for their role, and seek to gain more credibility through undertaking widely recognised courses (Atkin *et al.*, 1993), of which the RCN's nurse practitioner course is just one. Others (and many other community nursing staff) recognise that, with the pressures on the GP and the increasing workload facing the team, they could constructively expand their role to meet the needs of the community more appropriately. Again, the 'nurse practitioner' label is often used by them, yet their expectations and initial skill-base may be very different. This can lead to confusion not only for patients receiving care, but also for colleagues working alongside them. Who should they see? Who might they refer and where? What are the boundaries of their activity?

Complicating matters further, the UKCC has as yet only begun to consider what in fact it means by advanced practice, and how far that might overlap with some of the work of a range of other disciplines. To date it appears that advanced practice will be a relatively rare (and short-term) entry on the Nursing Register, assessed by a group of the practitioner's peers, and that it will depend not on academic prowess but on demonstrably high-level nursing skills, including an ability to set practice in a policy context, and also to develop and guide colleagues.

The term 'nurse practitioner' has been (mis)used to identify someone with specialist skills in a community setting – yet all community health care nurses are 'specialist nurses' according to the UKCC. Many so-called nurse practitioners could more accurately be called clinical nurse specialists. In Stilwell's original work, and in the USA, a generic remit was central to the role. The focus of most longer term posts has been on a wide-ranging approach to physical health. However, one area which has begun to expand in the USA (McConnell *et al.*, 1992), and which has been discussed in the UK (Torn and McNichol, 1996), is the mental health 'nurse practitioner' role. The changing direction of community psychiatric nursing to take on more serious and enduring mental health problems (Department of Health, 1994) may open the door for the further development of the mental health 'nurse practitioner' role in primary health care in the UK. One such experiment is already in place (Vardy, 1996), and more may follow. Systematic evaluation will be needed, which should incorporate the impact of such developments on other members of the team.

Nurse prescribing is mentioned only briefly in the White Paper. However, having been initially piloted in eight fundholding demonstration sites, it is currently (in 1996) being further piloted in Bolton Community Healthcare Trust, and should thereafter be 'rolled out' generally. It has the potential to generate either harmony or conflict within a primary health care team, since the costs of prescriptions will be charged back to the practice. There may be disagreement about the appropriateness of what has been prescribed, particularly if it is relatively expensive. If communication within the team is poor, there may also be little mutual understanding of priorities. However, if clear standards for prescribing have been agreed in relevant areas, problems are less likely to arise.

Among the most significant policy shifts of recent years (see Chapter 1) has been the strategic shift of resources from secondary to primary care, and therefore the increased importance for service development and research of the primary/secondary care interface. A number of new or changed roles have resulted, each of which impacts on the boundaries of the primary health care team. To some extent, the impact of such roles is dependent upon whether they originated in primary or community care, or in hospital care. For example, many of the early 'hospital at home' schemes were initiated by hospital staff, who were concerned to discharge patients home earlier. However, these schemes often experienced problems in communication with GPs and community nurses, and some were later transferred to management by community trusts. Rapid response teams are a more recent phenomenon, developed by community trusts in order to maintain patients at home and to avoid unnecessary admissions to hospital (Earl-Slater, 1995). They have not in general had difficulties in relating to primary care, but have not always been well understood in hospital settings. Further understanding is needed of roles originating in both areas of practice, and of their impact on care by colleagues.

One might also ask whether it is possible for primary care to cope. Do practitioners have the appropriate skills, and are sufficient resources being moved to primary care? The pressures that are developing from the strategic shift into primary care include, for example, greater expectation of medical, nursing and other staff to cover for people in residential and nursing homes, with few additional resources. Strategies for dealing with this have included the identification of a list of 'core' services – a minimum list which should always be provided – by medical negotiators, and the development of much tighter contracts by Health Authorities.

When looking at multidisciplinary working across the primary/secondary care interface, the other important factor to be considered is the organisational complexity involved. In recent work by the author on patient discharge, in which the records of individual patients were tracked across the interface, individual gatekeepers to different agencies or professional groupings were contacted. The implication of this is the need for discussions of teamwork in primary health care in order to draw on a broader definition of team, such as that advanced by Edward in Chapter 4. Where indeed are the boundaries?

Care in the Community developments (Department of Health, 1990) have also influenced patterns of working across and between disciplines. The boundaries between health and social care – always an area of contention – have become, in a range of pilot projects, subject to shared decision-making. The boundaries of practice between GPs, nurses and social workers are being explored, with development of greater understanding of roles, and of the criteria used to assess both health and social need. The views of the patients receiving such integrated services are also being examined. Further work is required to develop knowledge in this area.

The vision

What can we predict for the future, and what are the implications of that vision for research agendas? I believe that primary health care in the future will see a further expansion of the roles of nursing and the professions allied to medicine relative to GPs. Existing models of funding will move towards development of an integrated contract-based approach, with salaried GPs or mixed-discipline practice partnerships. Primary health care will be provided by a mixture of units, both GP-based groupings and groupings of nurses, health visitors, midwives and others (professions allied to medicine, social workers, etc.) to meet the needs of given localities, contracting into Health Authorities or groups of locality purchasers. Teams will thus be more broadly based and complex.

A range of specialist services will be provided to each locality through a local resource centre, with super-specialist services in some locations. These groupings will form teams that interface with more local primary care provision. Information systems will be moving towards becoming fully integrated, with every practitioner in primary care able to use a compatible system and to access epidemiological and other data routinely, in a user-friendly format. Communication in primary care will change, with the growth of effective electronic as well as face-to-face communication.

Nurses will increasingly be involved in work in minor injury and out-of-hours centres, developing skills in the sifting and management of self-limiting and minor health problems, whilst identifying and referring serious health problems. At the same time, the need for primary health care to be about maintaining *and* promoting health will be recognised. There will be increased emphasis on health promotion, especially primary prevention, community development and local public health work, much of which will be managed by nurses. Links with social care providers will be increasingly integrated within localities and at purchaser level, and social workers will play an increasing role in offering preventive care.

Primary care staff will, with patients' active participation, become the main managers of chronic disease, e.g. asthma, diabetes, arthritis care. Voluntary organisations will be seen as increasingly important, and will be integrated into care packages. As the number of older people in the community increases, the care of older people will become a major part of primary care. Collaboration between health and social care services will be essential in order to provide a 'seamless' service for patients. There will be access to an increased range of community-based resources (e.g. professions allied to medicine and geriatricians) in specialist, locality-based teams.

An increasing proportion of patients with long-term mental illness, especially those with anxiety and depression, will be dealt with by primary care, and innovative approaches to the management of this trend will be developed, with increasing emphasis on nursing-led approaches and on secondary and tertiary prevention.

Research into primary health care will be developing, providing a more robust evidence base for practice. Research training for practitioners of all disciplines in primary care will be developing at all levels, and will be actively encouraged. Existing trends to provide a greater proportion of undergraduate education for medicine and nursing in community contexts will be continued, with multidisciplinary teaching practices and groups developing.

Research agendas for the future

What research agendas arise from this vision with regard to teamwork in primary care? As evidence-based practice becomes less of an aspiration and more of a reality, there will be increasing demand for evidence both about organisational structures, processes and outcomes, and about practice itself. Practitioners need to know whether teamwork really does make a difference to patients. More studies will have to be undertaken on a sufficient scale to demonstrate change.

Most studies of primary health care teams, including those in this book, have failed to address the role of the patient in the primary health care team. The whole systems approaches favoured by McMaster University and the King's Fund may enable the primary health care team and its patients to be located in relation to one another, and to begin to explore some of the other impacts of the team's work. There is a need to explore such approaches, and to examine the feasibility and outcomes of community development approaches in health care.

The development of new organisational and contractual relationships between members of primary care teams and between teams and others will be another important area for research. Many organisational changes have been introduced previously with minimal attention to evaluation. The 1996 White Paper states that evaluation will be central to all pilot schemes. It will be crucial to look not only at outcomes for patients but also at issues such as power, decision-making and morale in reconfigured teams.

New roles – as well as the not so new, such as nurse practitioners – also require further exploration. This should include consideration of boundary disputes and territorialism between disciplines and agencies, questions about autonomy and decision-making at professional boundaries, examination of patients' perspectives on new roles, and investigation of colleagues' views and behaviour.

Nurse prescribing could also be treated in this way, looking at disputed territory, autonomy and decision-making. Research should look, for example, at debates about the appropriateness of what has been prescribed. Are the rationales advanced by GPs and nurses similar or different? Do nurses and doctors think differently? Is there a 'correct' answer, i.e. a standard? What do the patients think?

As further development takes place at the interface between primary and secondary care, well-designed evaluations are needed to examine the degree of integration of service achieved and the effect of different patterns of organisation (e.g. inreach or outreach). The organisational complexity involved must be captured, and the impact of this on the work of team members in primary care described.

Pilot projects promoting care management within primary health care settings and similar initiatives have encouraged practitioners in health and social care to test the boundaries between them. The boundaries between GPs, nurses and social workers have been subject to change and development. Research is needed on the impact of different organisational and contractual arrangements, methods of shared decision-making, ways of promoting understanding of roles between practitioners in health and social care, and criteria for assessment of both health and social need. The views of patients should also be sought.

Editors' summary

In this chapter, Pearson has set out some of the key influences which are likely to impact on the continuing development of multidisciplinary teamwork in primary health care, and she has developed a vision of what lies ahead. From this, she has identified the important agendas which research must address in the future. At the very minimum, if we are to encourage more integrated provision of primary health care across a range of agencies and disciplines, teamwork will be required. If teamwork is to be effective, then it must be planned and carried out from a strong research base. Only then will we be able to provide the highest quality health care for people and the communities in which they live.

References

Atkin K, Lunt N, Parker G and Hirst M (1993) *Nurses Count: A National Census of Practice Nurses.* Social Policy Research Unit, University of York.

Boyd M, Brummell K , Billingham K and Perkins E (1993) *The Public Health Post at Strelley: An Interim Report.* Nottingham Community Health NHS Trust, Nottingham.

Department of Health (1990) *Caring for People: Policy Guidance.* HMSO, London.

Department of Health (1994) *Review of Mental Health Nursing, Department of Health (the Butterworth Report).* Department of Health, London.

Department of Health and Social Services (1983) *NHS Management Enquiry (Griffiths Report).* Department of Health and Social Services, London.

Department of Health and the Welsh Office (1989) *General Practice in the National Health Service. A New Contract.* HMSO, London.

Earl-Slater A (1995) *An Economic Assessment of Coventry's Fast Response Service.* Health Services Management Centre, University of Birmingham, Birmingham.

Evans F (1987) *The Newcastle Community Midwifery Care Project: An Evaluation Report.* Newcastle Health Authority, Newcastle upon Tyne.

Grimshaw J and Russell I (1993) Effect of clinical guidelines on medical practice. A systematic review of rigorous evaluations. *Lancet* 342, 1317–22.

Jones K, Wilson A, Russell I *et al.* (1996) Evidence-based practice in primary care. *British Journal of Community Health Nursing* 1, 276–80.

McConnell S, Inderbitzin L and Pollard W (1992) Primary health care in the CMHC: a role for the nurse practitioner. *Hospital and Community Psychiatry* 43, 724–7.

National Health Service Executive (1996a) *Choice and Opportunity – Primary Care: The Future.* HMSO, London.

National Health Service Executive (1996b) *Primary Care: the Future.* Department of Health, Leeds.

Pietroni P and Chase HD (1993) Partners or partisans? Patient participation at Marylebone Health Centre. *British Journal of General Practice* 43, 341–4.

Ross FM, Bower PJ and Sibbald BS (1994) Practice nurses: characteristics, workload and training needs. *British Journal of General Practice* 44, 15–18.

Secretaries of State for Social Services, Wales, Northern Ireland and Scotland (1996) *Choice and Opportunity. Primary Care: the Future.* HMSO, London.

Stilwell B (1982) The nurse practitioner at work in primary care. *Nursing Times* 78, 1799–803.

Torn A and McNichol E (1996) Can a mental health nurse be a nurse practitioner? *Nursing Standard* 11, 39–44.

Vardy C (1996) *Nurse Practitioners in Mental Health: Dream or Reality?* Paper given at the Royal College of Nursing Nurse Practitioner Conference, Edinburgh, August 1996.

World Health Organization (1978) *Alma-Ata 1978. Primary Health Care: Report of the International Conference.* World Health Organization, Geneva.

Index

Page numbers printed in **bold** type refer to figures, those in *italic* to tables.